– Take the *"I don't have time to exercise"* challenge* –

The

I0084327

Zer⧗-Minute
Workout™

with

T✗eam™

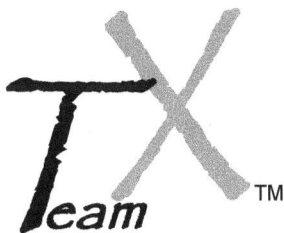

*using the techniques of an ✗er-task™

written by: Daniel Akin
(with Billy Nuzzo and Inara Lopetaite)

photographed by: John Graf
edited by: Dorothy Hilton

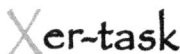

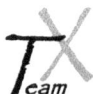

SOME WORDS OF ENCOURAGEMENT...

"It's never too late –
never too late to start over,
never too late to be happy."
– Jane Fonda

"All we have to decide
is what to do
with the time that is given us."
– J. R. R. Tolkien

"Don't let the fear of the time it will take
to accomplish something
stand in the way of your doing it.
The time will pass anyway;
we might just as well put that passing time
to the best possible use."
– Earl Nightingale

"There is no greater harm
than that of time wasted."
– Michelangelo

"Our greatest weakness lies in giving up.
The most certain way to succeed
is always to try just one more time."
– Thomas A. Edison

"Never, never, never give up."
– Winston Churchill

...SOME ENDORSEMENTS...

"I have known Billy Nuzzo for almost twenty years and like most people who've met him, I've always marveled at his physical conditioning and energy. The Zero-Minute Workout has distilled his years of nutritional knowledge and exercise experience into practical strategies and workouts that can be done at home or at work or almost anywhere.

As a Clinician, I find The Zero-Minute Workout to be an excellent guide for both diet and exercise and would encourage using the techniques in this book to all my patients, as an important step in integrating total fitness into their everyday life." – Jeffrey Farricelli, MD
Director, Center for Regenerative Medicine,
Charleston, SC

"The Zero-Minute Workout embraces the paradigm of combining easy, time-tested exercises with wasted time throughout the day. More than that, it provides a great recipe on how to reset your health for life by combining equal doses of exercise and dietary knowledge with a pinch of humor in an easy-to-follow program.

I would happily recommend The Zero-Minute Workout to my patients young and old." – C. Curtis Howard III, D.C.
Colonial Chiropractic, North Hollywood, CA

...AND SOME SELF-PROMOTION.

"People ask me all the time, 'Billy, how can I get a body like yours?' 'Cause I look in the mirror and even I can't look away. I like what I see. In fact if you don't like the way you look, then stop looking or do something about it. Stop admiring my butt and get off of yours! Work those glutes! Work those abs! Put down those donuts! 'Cause if you can't do that, then you don't really want a body like mine.

You need to stop staring, read this book and follow what I say. And don't tell me you don't have the time. You probably had time for pizza or fries the other day, right? Not for nothing, but, if The Zero-Minute Workout could change your life, would you have time for it then? Because it can." – Billy Nuzzo

"When I was a younger woman I used to eat what I wanted and without any thought to exercising. Now I know better. But working out, all starts with a proper diet.

We can't make you listen to us about getting in shape – as hard as Billy may try – but we can show you how. So, at the very least, look at the pictures in this book. If you like what you see, go for it. What do you have to lose?" – Inara Lopetaite

"Having known Billy for seventeen years, Inara for ten and observed their butts in person, I can vouch for both their structural and philosophical integrity. But I'll let the book speak for itself." – Daniel Akin

DEDICATIONS and ACKNOWLEDGEMENTS

I would have to say that my father was the first adult that inspired me with his wisdom, "What the f#@% are you working out for? Just do some hard work, that's all the exercise you will ever need. You're gonna die anyway just like everybody else!!!" I was 12-years-old at the time. If for no other reason than to protect myself from him, I did a 180 and immersed myself in martial arts, bodybuilding, and nutritional health. And I also learned the benefit of exercising throughout the day in everything I did. So, I give thanks and gratitude to all the people who've helped my mission of health and fitness or have just been an incredible influence in my life, both good and bad.

To my two, very good friends Danny Akin, and Tim James, who have always promoted me and helped keep me on track, so that one day... I appreciate you guys always being uplifting. And to the positive members of my family, thank you all for your support and acceptance, and forgiving me for being me.

To the hell-of-a-lot of people who come up to me almost daily and say, "What do you do to look that amazing?" "How can I look like you?" "Are you on some special diet?" "You can't be that old." – I thank them for all of their inadvertent support and ego boosts, especially on my down days, when a compliment or an irritating question was just the lift I needed. But not for nothing, what do you mean, "You can't be that old?"

To all the actors I've cooked for, coached, trained, and who've trusted me with their personal struggles, I thank you for listening and giving my thoughts and advice credence in a world of misinformation.

To my good friend, Dr. Jeff Farricelli – who, at his Beverly Hills clinic, listened and discussed all my revelations in fitness – I am grateful for all the solid feedback.

To my good friend, Ken Rohla – who introduced me to the world of raw veganism at a time when I was struggling with a health crisis – you completely changed my life. You took my health to a new dimension and assured me that our bodies were created to cure themselves if fed the right diet, and supplementation. I listened!! Western medicine let me down. Ken did not!!! Thank you Ken.

And lastly I thank myself for being so humble.

– Billy Nuzzo

* * * * * * * *

Growing up in Lithuania, under the rule of the former Soviet Union, I know a thing or two about struggle and the importance of gratitude for all that you have. Through the years of adversity, my parents taught me to take advantage of every opportunity to grow, even though my feet grew much faster than the size of my older sister's shoes. My family in Lithuania has been my biggest influence in everything I do, as is my new family in America.

I thank my two children for always giving me a reason to do better.

I thank my husband for his constant support and for encouraging every idea I have ever had – or at least telling me why it might not work and then helping me to find a way to make it happen.

To all my friends, pageant sisters and my fellow artists in the fields of fashion and entertainment, I thank you for making me try harder to be my best.

And with much gratitude, I have to thank Billy Nuzzo for a physique so close to perfection that I couldn't help but try to follow. – Inara Lopetaite

* * * * * * * *

When I was in the 5th grade, I started to write my first book. I never finished it. This work is dedicated to my younger self who still plans to finish it someday.

To Andy, Anne, Rick and Cindy who have always encouraged me to follow my inspirations; to Karin and Tom for kindly being there for me when I needed it most; to Billy and Tim James (and Ray Poblick, for nothing), my ever-friends and constant supporters; to my first family (every single one of you) for my childhood, my adulthood and for making me who I am; to Dottie Hilton for reading almost everything I have ever written and giving me her honest response, support and helpful suggestions, in writing and in life; and to Del Boy and Rodney (alter egos; soul mates; for who they represent) – I give my love, thanks and endless gratitude. I can never thank you all enough.

And finally, to Billy and Inara (and Dennis White) for being my inspiration – this book would not exist without you. – Daniel Akin

CONTENTS

– Section 1 –
Getting ready to Xer-task
(the what, how, why and when)

– Section 2 –
Doing the Xer-tasks
(individual exercises and exercise routines)

– Section 3 –

Xer-tasking for life
(incentives and tips to keep you going)

"People often say that motivation doesn't last. Well, neither does bathing - that's why we recommend it daily." – Zig Ziglar

FOREWORD

IT'S ABOUT TIME! Exercising for life is a mind-set and you've proven you have the desire simply by reading this. You've taken what just might be the first step toward a better you. And once you've acknowledged that you need help getting in shape, there's no use pretending any more that you don't. What you need now is the motivation to listen and begin. Because frankly, no one can do it for you.

Rest assured, The Zero-Minute Workout **is not** one of those intense workouts with unrealistic claims and expectations. **It is** a straight-forward, bare-bones program of simple exercises that work. With a fresh approach, it makes Old-School exercising new again.

The Zero-Minute Workout may sound like a contradiction of terms, but it's no gimmick. **Team** X takes fitness seriously, with the nutrition and exercising necessary to get there, but it also has a good time in its presentation. Like all things worthwhile The Zero-Minute Workout requires a degree of effort, but there's no reason it can't be an enjoyable journey. And **Team** X is here to help (and maybe push you a little along the way). You already have the time. So, go ahead. Enjoy the process! It's time to X**er-task!**

To paraphrase Sir Isaac Newton –

"A body at rest, stays at rest. But a body in motion... stays fit."

PREFACE

Back in the day, our ancestors got their exercise as part of their daily routine. Sadly, technology has made that practice almost obsolete.

The Zero-Minute Workout returns to basics by bringing exercise back to the task at hand. Using the simple method of **Xer-tasking**, it reestablishes exercise as a natural function in our daily regimen, by essentially using our time twice – like walking and chewing gum. While traditional workouts rely on timed routines, The Zero-Minute Workout presents a new/old way to exercise; a 24/7 circuit to get you started and keep you going with a healthier, energized lifestyle on a consistent basis. But it can only give you a framework for action. You will have to do the rest.

Admittedly, there is almost nothing new about the exercises contained in this book. It's the approach to exercising that's unique. The Zero-Minute Workout is structured to become part of your life, not something that you try to find time to do. It is meant to become something that's done automatically throughout your day. And although everyone is different, the basic rules are the same: if you have realistic fitness goals and are dedicated to the actions required, you will reach those goals.

There are loads of other workout programs available, many using DVDs. Some are worthwhile, but most profess results that are arguably unrealistic, with before and after photos that are often misleading and questionably typical. They appeal to our egos that want to look great in a swimming suit. But a tight, trim body isn't something you can buy, take out of a box and put on. It's an ongoing process that can be started any time and unfortunately stopped as quickly.

When you see one of those intense, workout videos – with sexy, energetic, ripped bodies in their mid-twenties or thirties, telling you, "You can do it" – it's motivating... for a while. But when a man in his late sixties and a woman in her early forties – both in amazing shape, tell you, "You can be fit at any age" – , that's not only motivating, it's impressive and inspiring... for life. To **Team** X that's success. And The Zero-Minute Workout, utilizing the benefits of Xer-tasking is designed to help you succeed in a practical manner.

NOTE: While you may want to get right to the exercises in the Section 2 chapter on Xer-tasking, we recommend that you read everything leading up to it. And you really shouldn't overlook Section 3 either. There is some good stuff in all of it. That said, for those who still can't wait, see Short Cuts – page 11.

"Coming together is a beginning; keeping together is progress; working together is success." – Henry Ford

MEET *Team* X

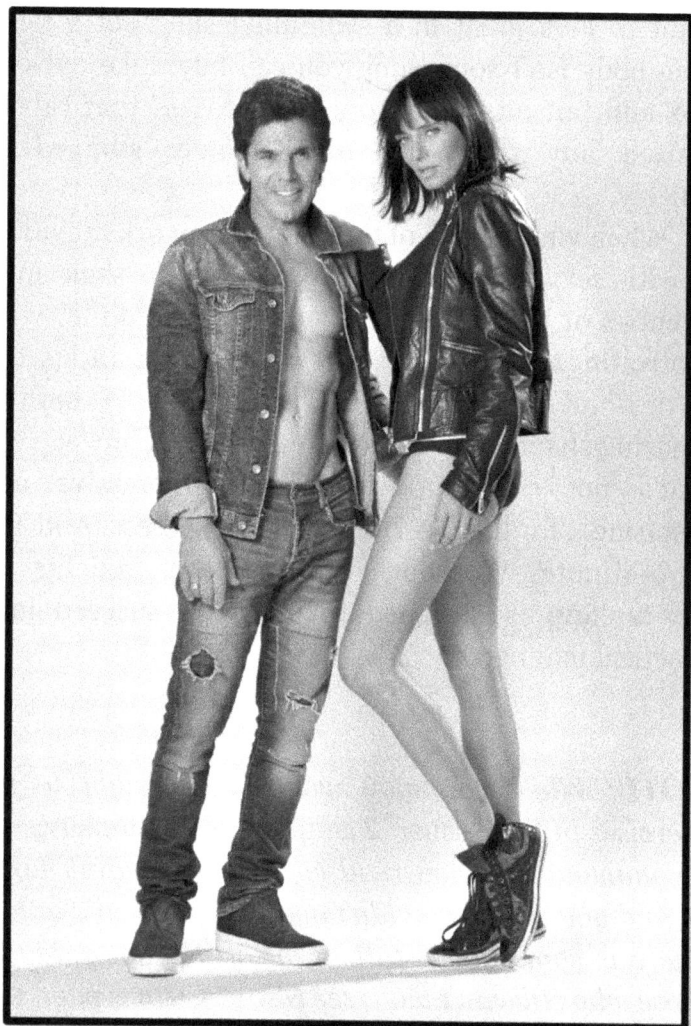

***Team* X** is Billy Nuzzo and Inara Lopetaite: two uniquely-qualified Fitness Coaches who've joined forces (with Daniel "Danny" Akin, as Co-Creator/ Writer) to share their knowledge so, along with your effort, dedication and persistence, you can be your best. They bring their expertise to the mat with the hope that an honest approach to exercising will be welcomed. Maybe it won't, but they don't know how to do it any other way and still feel good about themselves. Together, they have created The Zero-Minute Workout, combining various exercises with everyday activities (or inactivity) into an **X er-task,** to inspire the habit of exercising throughout each day.

***Team* X** was formed with a dedication to fitness and the science of exercising. And like all science there is a foundation of truth and a formula that must be followed to achieve the intended results. Looking good at 20 or even 35 is fairly easy. It's called, "youth". It's normal. Looking good and youthful – at 69 and 43, with pictures* to prove it – may not be normal, but it should be. And it can be that way for you, too.

*Unless otherwise noted, all pictures for this book were taken in 2014. This is just to acknowledge that while everyone presumably ages (except maybe Billy), that doesn't mean you have to slow down and certainly doesn't mean you should give up.

Billy and Inara (and even Danny) don't look the way they do because they're still kids. They look that way in spite of the fact they're not. And they're proud of that. They have the knowledge, the results and the age to back them up. Nothing is wrong with youth. We all want it. But if done right, age brings a few things that youth doesn't usually have: life experience, acquired wisdom and substantiated proof. In other words, **Team** X knows what they're talking about, because they've lived it (see the chapter, **MORE ABOUT Team** X, in Section 3 for additional info).

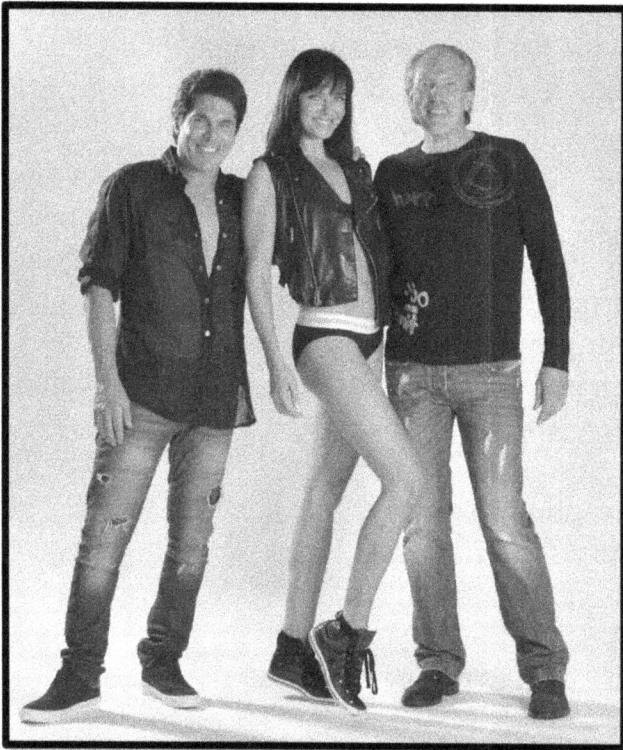

(Billy Nuzzo and Inara Lopetaite with Danny Akin)

– Section 1 –

Getting ready to Xer-task

(the what, how, why and when)

"Action is the fundamental key to all success." – Pablo Picasso

"I hated every minute of training, but I said, 'Don't quit. Suffer now and live the rest of your life as a champion'." – Muhammad Ali

INTRODUCTION

The Zero-Minute Workout shares or trades the same time that you are generally already using - doing something else - with an exercise or an exercise routine. It's a practical technique we call, **Xer-tasking** – a little hard to say, but fairly easy to do.

So much of our days are spent in passive activities that could easily share or even exchange their minutes with a better use of our muscles. Or our lives are spent waiting; waiting in traffic, waiting in line, waiting for a pot to boil, simply waiting and wasting time. Why not use our time better? Or use it again? The Zero-Minute Workout utilizes those static moments with exercises that are initially isometric (clenching the muscles, generally without moving them) and progresses on to isokinetic (tensing the muscles with controlled movement and resistance). An **Xer-task** relies on exercises that can provide the most benefits by either piggybacking on or substituting for the time another task is already using; exercises and routines you can do throughout your day or night, practically anywhere – either as a stand-alone program or as a supplement to an existing workout regimen you are already doing.

3

The Zero-Minute Workout is not like those insanely, rigorous workouts that you see so often on TV. If you can do them, great. The problem is, most people can't and we're not asking you to. In fact, The Zero-Minute Workout doesn't claim to get you ripped from head to toe in 90 days. It probably won't give you washboard abs in a month of 25-minute workouts or help you lose 21 pounds in 21 days. Some things just aren't possible. Though, all those young TV bodies eagerly sweating their way to perfection, may tempt us to try their exercise programs, are they practical... or truthful? Generally speaking, probably not. For most people, even if they can exercise at such a high energy level, they probably can't keep it up long enough to achieve the professed results. Getting ripped may not be for everyone. But wouldn't it be nice to get in better shape, if not just for your self-esteem? The results can literally be life-altering. But regardless of how you choose to get in shape, there isn't any way around it: *keeping fit and staying fit take a lifetime of devotion.*

If you're of the mind that exercise is too much work, then there is nothing anyone can do. But if you're ready, **Team** X can help. And realistically, isn't help in getting started – and to keep going – what you need? Because there are no miracle exercise routines – no machines or contraptions that will do the work for you – regardless of infomercial claims. In fact, no gyms or exercise machines are required. The only trick is, *you* have to do it. It's up to you to stick with it, but first you must make the decision to begin.

No matter the workout regimen, how fit you are now and how fit you decide to remain will take effort, dedication and persistence. Being in shape really isn't hard. It actually makes your life much easier. Being out of shape is quite simple, though it makes your life more difficult than it needs to be. In the end, there is only you and your life and what you make of it. Exercising can be a chore or it can be natural. So, why not enjoy the process? Of course not everyone is going to look like a super model, but the only look you should be going for anyway is a super you.

The Zero-Minute Workout is here to help, with no outrageous claims, just an honest, daily approach to exercising and getting fit with individual exercises and workout routines that are simple, practical and effective. Whether you are 14 or 104 (and approved by a physician to exercise) you can improve and maintain your fitness with determination and the right motion and activity; the right Xer-task. On that *Team* X guarantees.

"Step by step the thing is done." – Charles Atlas

1   BEFORE YOU BEGIN

The Zero-Minute Workout contains the following:

STAGE 1 (Individual Exercises)
LEVEL I: Muscle Training
LEVEL II: Muscle Movement
LEVEL III: Muscle Resistance

STAGE 2 (Beginning Exercise Routines)
Workout suggestions to get you started from exercises in LEVEL I: Muscle Training.

STAGE 3 (Intermediate Exercise Routines)
Workout suggestions to shake things up from exercises in LEVEL II: Muscle Movement.

STAGE 4 (Advanced Exercise Routines)
Workout suggestions for extra visible results from exercises in LEVEL III: Muscle Resistance.

STAGE 1 involves three levels of individual exercises that can be done throughout your day, at your own pace, whenever you choose.

STAGE 2, STAGE 3 and STAGE 4 involve individual exercise routines using the exercises of STAGE 1. They're structured to get you moving at a pace with which you can see increasing results yet won't wear you out in the process. Some may take more time management than others, simply requiring you to be a little more creative as you **Xer-task**.

Again, an **Xer-task** is an exercise or exercise routine you can do safely, at the same time you're doing something else or by swapping the time altogether with a task you might not need to do at all.

The Zero-Minute Workout shows you how you can exercise correctly, even when you thought you didn't have the time. It's designed to get you going with a new mind-set; to make exercising a part of your life; to get you into the habit of thinking...

> *"What can I do right now, that will keep me (or get me) in shape? In fact, I'm always thinking about how I can turn something into a workout. It started when I was a little kid running numbers for my Uncle Dickie. Now, even without a Bookie breathing down my neck I still do things like run up the stairs and quick curls with the groceries from the car to the kitchen. Stuff like that. It's habit with me now."* – Billy

Being out of shape with a poor eating routine is also a matter of habit. Just as is being in shape. Which habit do you want to create? What lifestyle pattern are you going to follow? If you've programed yourself to be lazy, to take the easy way, to eat greasy foods, to say, "I don't want to exercise", the only conclusion you can come to is an unhealthy lifestyle. But if you program yourself to try a little harder, eat a little healthier, give a little more effort, then your body will improve. It has to. But to achieve it, you first must visualize it.

Visualization starts with seeing yourself as the best you can be. This isn't the same as accepting an out of shape body as your best. It's holding to the best image of yourself that you can imagine. You must set your course for healthier horizons in order to reach them. If you lose sight of those goals you may not ever get to where you originally wanted to go. You will however, get to where you ended up "not planning" to go.

If we don't set our sights on a better, healthier, more-fit life, chances are we won't achieve it. Our muscles won't get there on their own. We must first tell them what we expect by programming a better life as our self-image default. We must make it a habit.

The Zero-Minute Workout was created to give you the right habits, with exercises you can do throughout your day. Once exercising becomes routine, it's easier to move on to – or continue with – longer, more involved workouts. In fact, one of the problems with most workout programs is they usually ask too much. For someone who isn't used to exercising, the idea of a daily twenty to thirty minute workout can be daunting and actually attempting to do it may be the very thing that erroneously convinces you that you can't.

People who are in great shape generally didn't just start off exercising rigorously. They worked up to it. Long distance runners don't start off running twenty miles at a clip. Bodybuilders don't start by lifting four hundred pounds over their heads. And you shouldn't start with an exhausting, full workout either. A full commitment, yes.

One of the easiest things to start with is to walk. But we don't mean stroll. This is not about leisure; it's about what's best for your health. And unless a Doctor has advised you otherwise, walking is great for your health. Walk everywhere that you can but walk briskly. Walk with a purpose; the purpose to lose any excess weight you may have. Walking can not only help you lose weight, it will increase your heart rate and regulate your blood flow. And if you can safely run instead, then run. You don't have to sprint but a good trot now and then is invigorating.

In other words, start moving and keep moving. Because our bodies basically have two choices – to be at rest or to be in motion. Of course we can't always be moving. Sometimes rest is good. Everybody needs it, sometimes. But the rest of the time... choose motion. When you have the chance to activate your muscles... then choose motion. You can simply watch TV or you can turn your viewing into an **Xer-task**. You can wait in line at a store or **Xer-task** your way to the check-out. You can let the elevator raise you up or elevate your heart rate by walking up the stairs instead. You can even run up if you want, just maybe not in heels.

The idea is for **Xer-tasking** to become second nature. Because once keeping fit, healthy and energetic becomes habit in your head, your body will follow. It has no choice. So choose wisely. Choose exercises or routines that are practical for you right where you are – ones that will get you ready for the next step. Then keep stepping.

And while you have your legs moving, you might want to try out a bicycle. It's a great workout for your heart, quads, butt, calves, triceps and your abs. Again, don't go crazy. Set your distance goals on mileage you can reach, realizing that you have to come back.

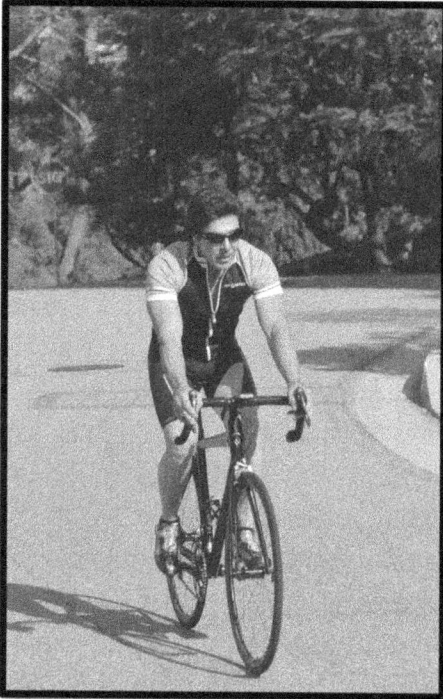

"The science of exercise is beautiful. And so are the results. I've been riding about 45 miles, two or three times a week, for the last ten years. And frankly, that's not the usual motion for a 69 year old. But it should be."
– Billy

(In other words, you can do it. Just try.)

NOTE: *When doing a daily workout or individual exercise, unless it's a large muscle like the butt or stomach or you're doing aerobics or whole body moves, it's best to vary the muscles used. Do an arms day, a legs day, a chest day, a whole body day, etc. In other words, remember to work your whole body but if you do muscles like arms or legs one day don't do them the very next day. Muscles need time to recover.*

Short Cuts: If you're still looking for short cuts to fitness, we hate to tell you, there aren't any. No matter what some infomercials claim, they simply don't exist. However, here are a few short cuts for this book for people like Billy (and even Inara) who just can't wait.

– Section 2 –

1) At the end of each level in STAGE 1 are lists of **Daily/Weekly Exercise Suggestions**. If you do no other exercises, at least try to do the following:

LEVEL I: Muscle Training – pg. 76
LEVEL II: Muscle Movement – pg. 131
LEVEL III: Muscle Resistance – pg. 194

2) STAGE 2, STAGE 3 AND STAGE 4 are comprised of suggested workout routines using the individual exercises of the three increasingly difficult levels in STAGE 1, organized by specific muscles and muscle groups as follows:

STAGE 2 (LEVEL I – Beginner) – pg. 197
STAGE 3 (LEVEL II – Intermediate) – pg. 212
STAGE 4 (LEVEL III – Advanced) – pg. 230

– Section 3 –

3) And lastly, here is some additional, individual info and stats about who you're dealing with.

THINGS WE EAT – pg. 266
MORE ABOUT *Team* X – page 294

Now stop your stalling and move forward.

"The only way you get that fat off is to eat less and exercise more." – Jack LaLanne

"Being entirely honest with oneself is a good exercise." – Sigmund Freud

2 WEIGHING THE TRUTH

This is not the time to be politically correct. The truth is what matters here. Like it or not we must talk about the elephant in the room – the one that most people don't want to discuss – and that elephant is, "fat".

There are many levels of being fat. Some people are just slightly overweight, while others are genuinely obese. Regardless, if your body has excess fat and you want to get rid of it, then you have to acknowledge the fat. There is nothing wrong with loving yourself as a person, in whatever state you are in. We recommend it. It's a healthy state of being. But if you are going to love the fat, then you will probably keep the fat. You have to make up your mind. Fat or fit? The fact is, you can't be both. It may help your self-esteem to think you can, but you can't. And if you really want to help your self-esteem and especially your health, you'll start taking steps to lose the weight. In fact, take the steps, literally. Take the stairs, walk, run, anything that gets your body moving on your own accord from here to there. But as important as exercise is, eating right may be even more so and there is no denying it.

It simply can't be emphasized enough that, <u>if you honestly want to get in shape with a healthier life then you are going to have to lose most of the excess fat</u>, especially if muscle definition is your goal. And the best way to start losing fat is to change your eating habits. You need to make a change that you can stick with, at your own pace; something you can do without the stress of severe dieting. Diets only really work if you do them willingly. If you're always thinking about food, either you aren't dieting willingly or you have the wrong diet or both. In fact, we aren't even going to suggest a particular diet program. Not yet anyway. We are, however, strongly suggesting that you eat healthier and exercise more – right now. If you do, the body will respond and flourish. Just start. You can always do better as you go. We will try to guide you. It's up to you to follow.

To start, eating right generally begins when you stop eating wrong. And for most people that will also mean unlearning a lifetime of bad eating habits. Now, before you panic, this is probably not something you can undo in a day, a week or even a month. So, don't try unless that's what you really want to do. Because that's not what we're asking you to do. In fact, you don't have to do anything we tell you. You don't even have to eat less. But if you are overweight and you want to look better in your clothes, then you absolutely must start eating better and start losing the fat now. There is no way around it. Again, fat and fit aren't the same! They are not compatible... period!

In most cases, our fat means we eat too many bad carbohydrates (see **GOOD CARBS vs BAD CARBS** at the end of the Section 3 chapter, **THINGS WE EAT**). Understanding how to eat right and get rid of the fat can be complicated, but it's worth learning.

Without getting too technical, ingested sugar is converted into glucose, which insulin then stores in the liver. When sugar exceeds the storage capacity of the liver it's converted into fatty acids, returned to the bloodstream and distributed throughout the body as fat, to all those places we see the most: the waist, butt, thighs and breasts. Then, once those fat cells are full, the fatty acids overflow into our organs, like the heart, liver and kidneys. And that's not a good thing.

Here is the too-often scenario. When our insulin level gets too high, from excess sugar, our body's fat-burning process shuts down, which means only the just-ingested sugar is used and delivered to the muscles. As soon as their storage is full the excess sugar is converted to fat and stored in our waistline. The insulin levels then drop causing our blood sugar levels to drop, causing our appetite to increase, causing us to want to eat more, which causes the whole process to start all over again.

Simply put: in order to burn fat, instead of sugar, STOP EATING PROCESSED SUGAR AND OTHER BAD CARBS, AND EXERCISE MORE (especially whole-body exercises – targeted exercises build muscle but don't really diminish fat). Doing it is easier than explaining it, but in a nut shell, that's it.

The truth is, though, everyone has good days and bad. Weights and diets fluctuate and either we don't always feel like exercising or eating right or our bodies are simply changing. It happens to all of us – even Billy (who constantly alters his diet and routine), Inara (who's been known to need a restart) and Danny (always). But the difference between a healthy, fit life and one that's not is that when someone with a practical map for a healthy life falters, they get back on the path (treadmill, bicycle, etc.) and pick up the pace. And that's the idea that **Team** X represents.

It's beyond the scope of this book to lay out a total dietary and nutritional plan, though one may be in the future from **Team** X. For now, at least try the following suggestions and check out the chapter, **THINGS WE EAT,** for a few helpful recipes.

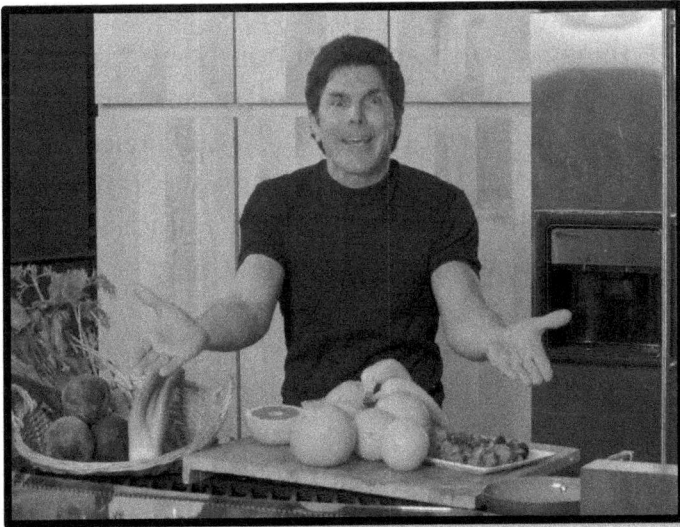

(Billy's plea may be pathetic, but at least it's earnest.)

SUGGESTION #1: Whatever unhealthy or fattening things you're eating, eat less of them.

Do you really need every one of those French fries? Maybe you could leave a few. Maybe you don't need to supersize your lunch today. Maybe one and a half slices of pizza might be enough instead of two. Maybe that extra helping of mashed potatoes and accompanying gravy aren't really that necessary. Just because you see food doesn't mean you have to eat it.

Anyway, we think you get the picture. It all adds up and as far as your weight is concerned, thankfully, so does every ounce we lose.

SUGGESTION #2: Try cutting out added sugar and other bad carbs and salt.

These may be the toughest things for you to give up. Let's face it, most of us love sugar and most everything we eat has way too much salt. Salt retains water weight, and many carbs – besides being wasted calories – only turn to excess sugar and hence, fat.

Letting go of the salt will probably be the easiest thing to do. Sea salt is healthier than processed or you can try an imitation salt if you have to have it. There's already so much salt in most processed foods (which we recommend you eat as little of as possible) and if you are using butter (which we recommend you cut back on) the salted variety has more than enough. And finally, instead of salted butter, you could switch to unsalted (see **Suggested Substitutions** at the end the chapter, **THINGS WE EAT**).

Cutting back on added/processed sugar and other bad carbs* is probably going to be your biggest challenge. They raise our energy levels like drugs, because they are. As high as we go, we come crashing down, just as far. But we're not suggesting you give up carbs altogether. Our bodies need a certain amount of carbs, so we recommend you cut back on them slowly in order to find a comfortable balance. Pure sugar (sucrose), on the other hand, is as useless for our wellbeing as things can be. We suggest you research the complex subjects of carbs and sugars, for yourself, on how their intake affects our bodies. You might also want to read diet books such as Atkins, which can be beneficial and good sources for low-carb/low sugar dieting and are much more in-depth than this book.

Unfortunately, sugar is added to so many things that you may not realize how much you are ingesting. Take a look at the food labels next time. You might be amazed at how many products contain added sugar. While you're looking, check the percentage of carbs and choose products with the least. Whatever you decide, do it in a way you can handle, without being so drastic you want to quit. And if you do have a set-back, don't worry. It's all a process. Just don't give up.

*see **GOOD CARBS vs BAD CARBS** in the chapter, **THINGS WE EAT**, because it's important to know the difference and that good carbs do exist. Billy's diet is full of good carbs, Inara's diet generally avoids the bad and Danny's diet... well he tries.

SUGGESTION #3: Monitor the amount of sodas and alcohol that you drink.

Like giving up pure sugar and cutting back on other carbs, reducing the intake of your favorite cola or night cap may be much easier said than done. Then again, it might just be easier to do than you think, but you won't know until you try. And it's worth trying.

Sodas and alcohol are fairly compelling to a body that's made them part of its daily routine, possibly for decades, so don't get discouraged. But our major concern is the amount of sugar they contain. Beer bellies could easily be called sugar bellies. And not much gives you a sugar high faster than a soft drink, which most times could easily be called a sugar drink.

If soft drinks are your thing, then you could cut back or switch to one with zero calories (diet sodas have their own problems but that's not what we're discussing here) or try seltzer. Or best yet, drink water instead. It quenches your thirst and benefits the body.

"I wouldn't ever touch a soda. Just saying." – Billy

If you like to drink alcohol, at least cut back. This isn't a guilt thing, it's a fitness thing. Alcohol simply isn't conducive to a healthy workout. And next time you're thinking about getting loaded, remember that wine and beer are loaded with sugar. We aren't even going to try to convince you to have a glass of water instead of an ice-cold brewsky. Just think about what the added sugar is doing to your waistline. Maybe that will be all the incentive you need to cut back (or stop).

SUGGESTION #4: Start eating healthier (and make, *"when you're ready"* <u>now</u>).

Starting an exercise program and going on a diet at the same time can be an almost impossible scenario to comprehend, let alone accomplish. So, be kind to yourself. We aren't asking you to do anything drastic. Just try some changes, as quickly as you feel comfortable in doing so. Hopefully sooner than later.

Cutting back on salt, processed sugar and other bad carbs is already a major step in the process of losing weight and regaining your rightful physique. Eliminating them totally is best, so do what you can. But there are additional healthier choices you can make when it comes to what you put into your system, such as eating more fruits and vegetables, which also happen to generally be among the good carbs. Most vegetables are great sources of the fiber we need for proper digestion and while fruits contain fructose (a natural form of sugar) it's an energy booster that unlike processed sugars and honey doesn't turn to fat, with a few exceptions*.

Again, you'll find some recipes for healthy eating (Billy's), healthier eating (Inara's) and fairly healthy eating (Danny's) in the chapter, **THINGS WE EAT**.

*Pineapples, grapes, bananas and others contain high amounts of fructose. Limited consumption is advised. (see **GOOD CARBS vs BAD CARBS** in the chapter, **THINGS WE EAT** for a fuller explanation.)

"If we could give every individual the right amount of nourishment and exercise, not too little and not too much, we would have found the safest way to health." – Hippocrates

3   GETTING STARTED

Assuming you've begun to eat right or you're at least trying, then you're ready to get started with an exercise program you can stick with. But in addition to a proper diet you should also be aware of the four phases to the proper exercising of your muscles.

1) **Contract** – move a muscle from its normal relaxed position.

2) **Engage** (fully) – tense a muscle as hard as you possibly can.*

3) **Visualize** – picture the muscle being engaged in your mind or if in front of a mirror, watch the movement.

4) **Release** – slowly stop the tensing of a muscle.

* Tensing a muscle does not mean straining a muscle. Caution is advised when lifting any weights, using machines, or applying resistance of any kind.

WARNING: For many Xer-tasks it may not be possible or even wise to visualize the muscle being worked (i.e. while driving a car; using a knife; an activity where most of your attention is required).

Most people use only two phases of exercising: Contract and Release. Yet by so doing they're cheating themselves out of the full benefit of an exercise. When you perform any movement at all, your muscles contract automatically, but they don't automatically fully engage. And although you're most likely aware of the main muscles you're using, being aware is not the same as visualizing those muscles being worked and growing bigger. The brain will always pick the easiest muscles to work an exercise. Fight it. That's what actively visualizing specific muscles helps you to do.

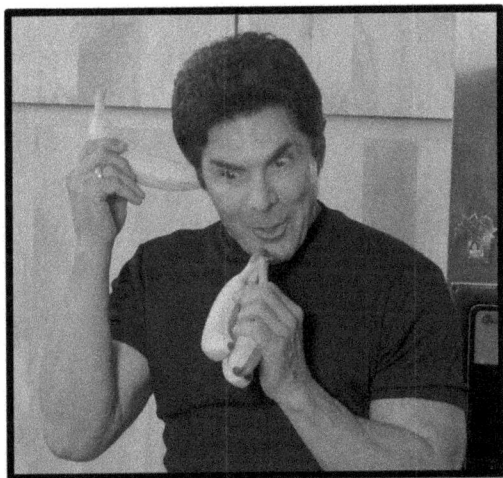

"I talk to my muscles. In fact, I swear at 'em and even threaten 'em, that if they don't grow I'll beat 'em. That's just me. But not for nothing..."
— Billy

NOTE: *Admittedly, you probably can't literally talk to your muscles through a banana, however, fruit and vegetables do connect directly with your muscles by the nutriments they provide. So, in a way, you're talking to them each time you eat healthy. That said, pretending to actually have a conversation on a banana phone is just a bit on the whacky side.*

Remember, if you want to truly benefit from an exercise you must do your best to Contract, Engage (fully), Visualize and then Release. Try to make this a habit and you'll absolutely see the results in your muscle tone. And one way to fully engage a muscle is to do an isometric exercise. We often do isometrics without realizing it, such as when we clench and hold a particular muscle at the end of a set.

Try this: while holding the back of a chair for balance, lift one leg backwards and up. Hold it in place a few seconds, release and lower it back. Now, lift the same leg again, this time, clenching the muscles on that side of your butt and the back of your leg as hard as you can. Picture the muscles you're squeezing; see them tightening. Feel the difference? You should, unless you aren't clenching hard enough or you've already learned the proper way to do it. To be sure, try squeezing that same side of your butt again, as hard as you possibly can. Remember how that feels, because during The Zero-Minute Workout you are going to be doing a lot of butt squeezing. Your own that is.

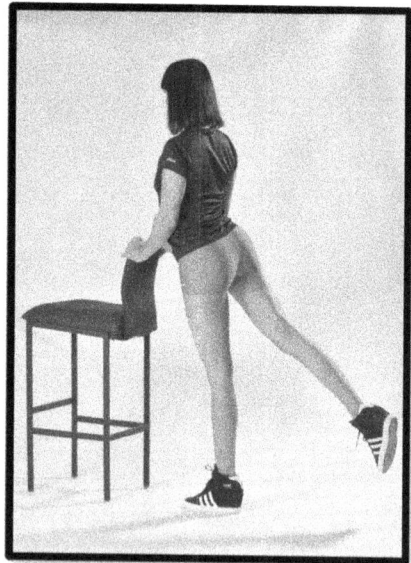

As you begin, you might find it helpful to keep a journal of each exercise that you did that day, so you'll know what's working for you and what isn't. We recommend you switch things up a little from time to time and don't always do the same exercises. You can work the same muscle groups (alternating days for smaller muscles) but work them using a different exercise. If you get too used to an exercise, you're more apt to not give a little more and so slow your progress. Also, try varying the degree of intensity of your exercising. For example, you could do bursts of several sets of push-ups as fast as you can one day, and at your regular pace, the next. The same can be done with workout routines. Simply vary the intensity and the exact exercises involved. Our bodies have well over 600 different muscles. Obviously, the same five or so different exercises won't quite be enough. But it's a start. So don't stop.

NOTE: *Throughout the exercises, we often refer to a particular "count" – the number of reps (repetitions; movements) and the number of sets of reps we suggest you perform or the amount of time* to do them. You can alter the amount of reps and sets to your liking, however, whatever number you choose it's best to stick with that amount so you will be able to gauge your progress effectively and alter either the time or resistance as needed.*

*When referring to time, use "one, one thousands", "two, one thousands", etc., as when counting seconds.

– Section 2 –

Doing the Xer-tasks

(individual exercises and exercise routines)

"I tell my sons all the time, 'The most important thing in your life is fitness,' but a lot of fighters go overboard."– George Foreman

4   Xer-tasking

If you're looking to bulk up or achieve muscle definition, you may not see it happen by **Xer-tasking** in STAGE 1 or STAGE 2 alone. While any exercise is better than none, for more results, more effort is required, probably going beyond STAGE 1 and STAGE 2 with longer blocks of shared or swapped time. To start, you'll need the routines of STAGE 3 and STAGE 4 that require more dedication, with specific groups of exercises, at least three to four times a week. That's not to say, STAGE 1 and STAGE 2 can't have a palpable effect, because they can. First they'll get you started and second, they should keep you going. But to gain more, you'll need to give more. The Zero-Minute Workout only works if you do it – as much as you can. Following the STAGE 3 and STAGE 4 exercise routines will have you well on your way to noticeable results. And if you're ready for them now, go for it. Otherwise, move on to STAGE 1.

NOTE: *Again, referenced reps or sets are suggestions only. Choose what works best for you.*

WARNING: Whenever using an elastic strap for resistance, always make sure it is secure. The sting of getting slapped isn't pleasant. (Billy knows this well.)

STAGE 1
(Individual Exercises)

Remember, all of the exercises in STAGE 1 are individual exercises and as such can be conducted whenever you think of doing them. If you can arrange your time to do several sets during a short session great, but you don't have to, although it's better if you do. That said, there is also a major benefit to be had from sporadically exercising here and there – the main thrust behind The Zero-Minute Workout: the habit of exercising throughout the day. By exercising with no particular large blocks of allocated time, you also may even find that you are completing more exercises than you would have, normally. However, don't ever let us stop you from finding ways to exercise more or longer. Whatever works for you.

At the end of each level you'll find **Daily/Weekly Exercise Suggestions** whether or not you do any of the others. Of course you're free to pick and choose exercises from whichever level you want to perform, but it's good to have an outline so you don't lose track of the goals you are trying to accomplish. Also, the following suggestions are helpful for every level.

1) Make a list of all of the exercises you plan on doing each day; legs, arms, chest, butt, stomach, whole body, and so on. It's too tempting to slack off, because chances are that's already your habit. The point is, to change your daily routine.

2) Do at least one exercise for the Butt and/or Stomach every day, preferably more. And try to increase that number ASAP.

3) If you know you are going to have certain times during the day when performing an Xer-task is going to be easy to do, then plan on it (i.e. coffee breaks; TV commercials; planes, trains and automobiles; etc.) Also plan on particular exercises that you want to do if and when an unplanned opportunity should occur (i.e. a long line at the store; a pot that never seems to boil; a TV show that it turns out you've already seen; etc.).

CAUTION: If you find that any of your muscles are cramping (especially the calves), immediately try to force the cramping muscle in the opposite direction, trying to stretch it back out. Then stop doing that movement for a while. Unless you like cramps. Either way, if you do cramp up, at least you'll know where the muscle is. But seriously, you don't want a cramp.

NOTE: *An* Xer-task *is the combination of a controlled movement (an exercise) and an activity (a task). By no means does* The Zero-Minute Workout *include every exercise there is.* **Team** X *has tried to put together a comprehensive list but it doesn't claim to include "the" definitive list of all the exercises possible – because that's not possible – but it is well-rounded. So, feel free to include any other movements that work for you with the activities of your choice.*

LEVEL I: Muscle Training

As we've said, there are no shortcuts to a better body and a healthier life. But there is a choice as to how quickly you want to get there. And the only way to do that is to start.

LEVEL I mainly involves isometric exercises with an occasional movement or resistance. Most can easily be conducted during your daily activities. It's an excellent place to begin; useful for anyone at any workout level because it helps remind us what really clenching a muscle feels like and when performed throughout the day keeps us in an exercising mode. If done right, you'll find that LEVEL I does a pretty good job of fatiguing your muscles, which may sound like something you don't want, but you do. The primary muscle groups worked out here are the stomach and butt, which happen to be most people's main problem areas. Other muscle groups are worked too, just not with quite the same degree of effectiveness, except for the chest and biceps which do react well to isometrics.

Research is finding that isometrics help to sculpt your body, promote lean muscle mass and increase your metabolism. In fact, The American Council on Exercise suggests that frequently performing small exercises – such as isometrics – will help increase calorie burning throughout your day. Additionally, isometrics are recognized as a relatively safe way to work your muscles during rehabilitation, with little stress or strain to the muscles and joints.

Depending on the isometric exercise, you might want to try doing them in three stages when possible, either in consecutive sets or on alternating days. Since isometrics are stationary, sometimes the only way to work the whole muscle is to clench it in different muscle lengths (i.e. for biceps: 1. Arms fully extended; 2. Bent halfway; 3. Bent all the way). Clenching the muscle a high number of times works to increase strength, while holding the clench longer works to increase mass. Just mix it up. Experiment with different positions to get the best overall results.

Nothing we are telling you in this book is new on its own. We are simply revealing a way to incorporate exercises into your life that can most benefit your health and fitness, starting with isometrics. Our plan here, as with all of **STAGE 1**, is to habitually incorporate individual exercises into your regular activities throughout your whole day, no matter your personal level of fitness or exercise routines.

WARNING: Isometric exercises tend to increase blood pressure and so may not be recommended for those individuals who already have high blood pressure. Always check with a Physician first.

Suggested Accessories*:
    Exercise mat, Yoga mat or soft rug
    Rope, soft strap, belt, old tie or elastic band
    Hand towel or cloth napkin

*It's your choice. Whatever works for you.

#1 THE BUTT (Gluteus Maximus or Glutes)

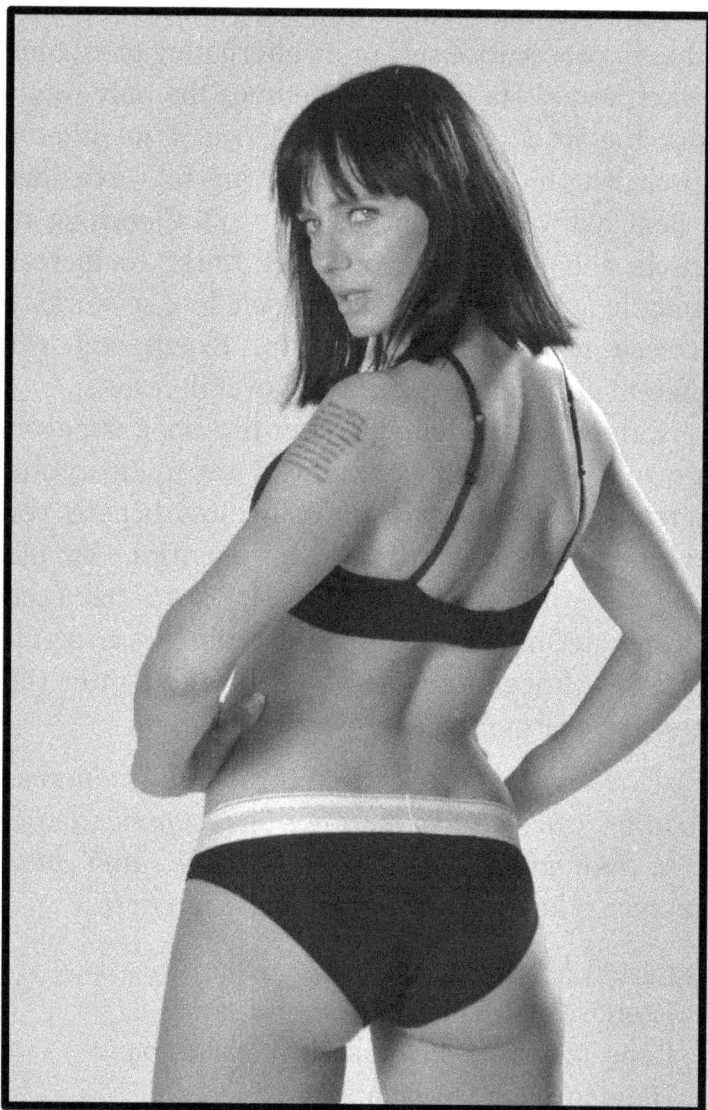

Our guess is, we don't have to point it out to you.

a) <u>Standing-Still Butt Clench</u>

This is an excellent exercise to do while standing in a line and waiting, because you can do this completely unnoticed by those around you. It's also something that can be done many times throughout the day, because the butt is one of those large muscles that you can't overwork too easily... and it won't hurt to try.

Clench one butt cheek (left pic) as hard as you absolutely can, trying not to engage any other muscle. Really visualize that muscle tightening up. Hold the clench. We mean really, really hold it, then release. Do this as many times as you can. Then do the same with the other cheek. Repeat if you're able. You'll feel it.

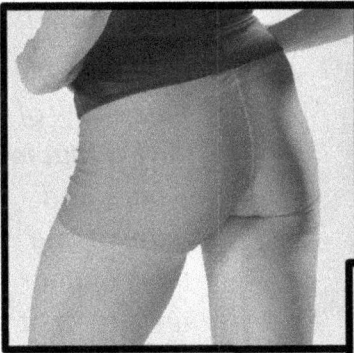

ALTERNATE VERSION: Standing on both legs evenly (right pic) clench from side to side or both cheeks together.

NOTE: *When clenching only one cheek at a time, keep your weight on the back leg – the one with the butt cheek being clenched.*

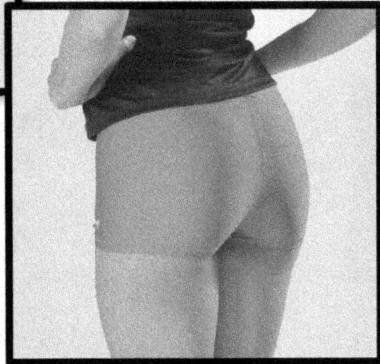

b) <u>Walking Butt Clench</u>

This exercise might take some getting used to. It is not powerwalking. It's more like "glutewalking". If you have to walk somewhere anyway, especially if it is a long distance, you might as well fully engage your butt cheeks and really get a workout. For every step you take, clench that cheek as hard as you can while moving forward. This will probably feel awkward at first and may look even sillier. But with a little practice you should find that your walk will look fairly normal, but the results can be way above normal.

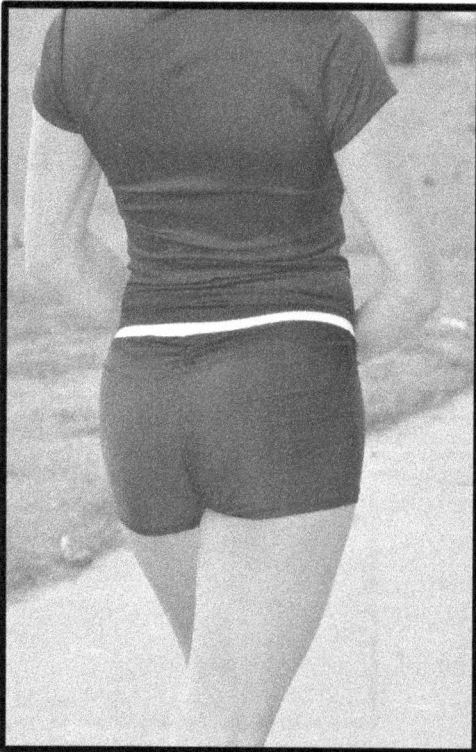

HINT: You should only be clenching the butt cheek of the leg that is back and supporting most of your weight – not the leg that is stepping forward – just as Inara is doing here.

c) <u>Butt Clench Squats</u>

This exercise is a good one to do while watching television or when you find yourself sitting and waiting for an extended length of time. Though doing this in a Doctor's waiting room might not be the best idea, unless you really want the attention.

Arch your back, stick your butt out, then with your feet about one foot apart*, squat down bending your knees, with arms forward and hold. Try hard to isolate your cheeks as you clench. Since this also works your thighs, lower back and hamstrings, it may take a bit of practice before you can feel it mainly in your glutes. Just do this as many times as you can.

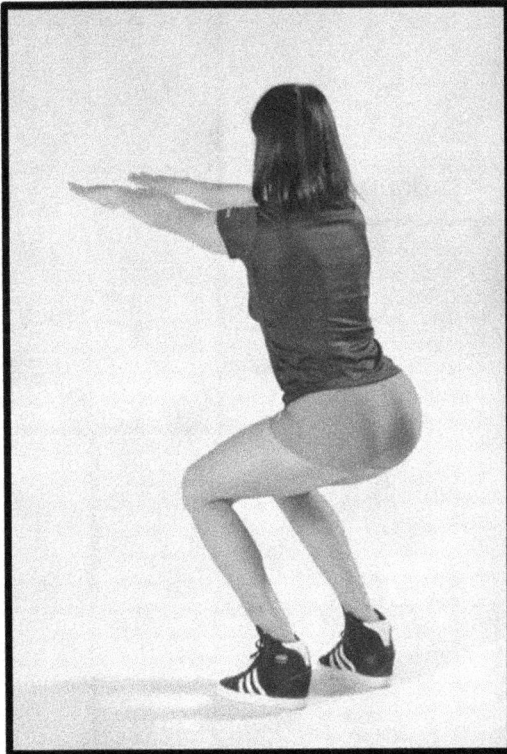

* The wider your feet (toes out) the less stress on your knees. If any pain, STOP.

d) <u>Standing Butt Clench Leg Lifts</u>

Raise one leg backwards, clenching that butt cheek and hamstring. Release and repeat. Do this as many times as you feel comfortable, with both legs. Then do it some more throughout the day whenever you can.

The *Freestanding* version is the easiest to do. No need for hands on your hips (that's Inara), just don't kick anyone. *Leaning* against a wall gives you a better lift. And *Balancing* is better still.

Leaning

Freestanding

Balancing

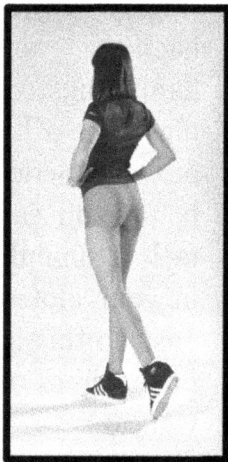

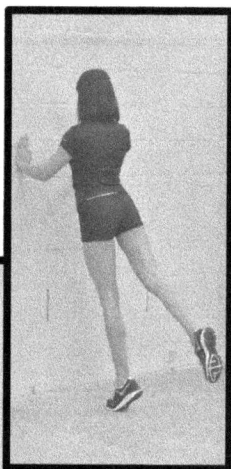

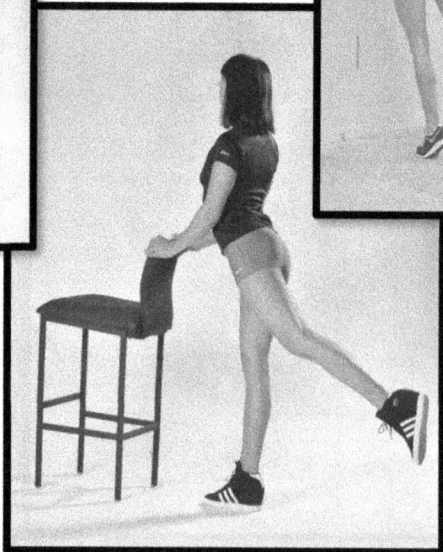

NOTE:
The higher the lift and the tighter the clench, the better the results.

e) <u>Chair Butt Clench</u>

Version #1: Using a chair, or any surface that won't push away, isolate and clench one butt cheek at a time. Hold for at least a five count and do as many reps as you can. Repeat again, when and if you're able.

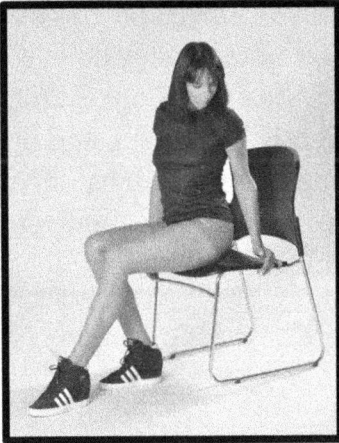

Version #2*: Hovering between the edge of a chair (or other secure surface) and the floor – supporting yourself from behind, with your legs bent about 90 degrees, as shown below – clench your butt and hamstrings, <u>trying not to use your thighs or triceps</u>. Hold for a five count and repeat until you can't. You might also want to try clenching at various heights.

WARNING: Never do Version #2 while driving, and if doing Version #1, use caution, especially if clenching for distance goals. A clench could engage your calves by mistake.

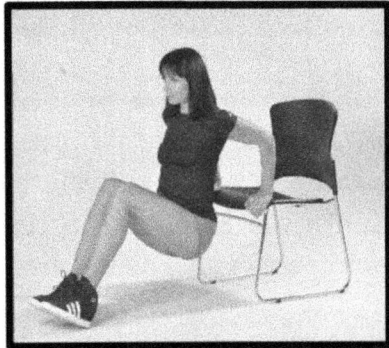

*(See LEVEL II: #1 BUTT and BACK LEG EXERCISES – c) Chair Squats, for a moving version.)

f) Lying-Down Leg-Lift Butt Clench

This clench involves the same move as the Standing Butt Clench Leg Lift, while lying on your stomach*. We also recommend a soft surface like a mat or a rug, or if you do them in bed, a firm mattress is best. Now we can think of other "exercises" to do in bed but this happens to be one you can easily do while doing something else, such as watching TV or reading.

Raise one leg at a time, slightly bent, back and up, while simultaneously clenching that leg's butt cheek and hamstring, for a five-count. Do this for a few reps each leg and on each last rep, clench and hold.

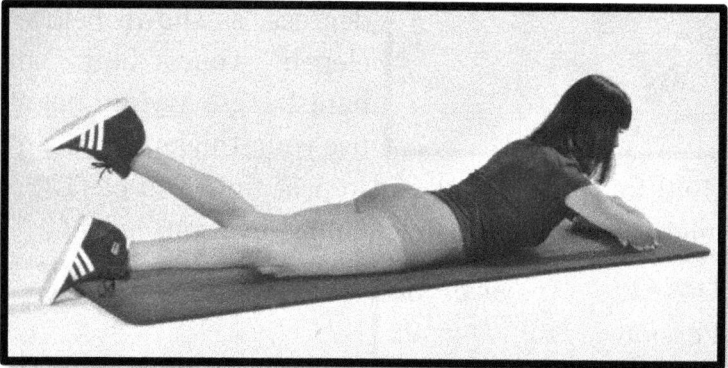

You can also try raising both legs at once – whatever way you feel the best results – because unlike the Standing Leg Lift version you can clench both cheeks at the same time.

*NOTE: Although Inara arches her back, the straighter you keep it the better. Also, a pillow under your hips can help reduce unwanted strain.

g) Sitting Hip Abductor Clench

This exercise works your glutes and outer thighs where they connect to your hips. It's perfect for the office at a desk (though a shirt might be a good idea).

While sitting, with your legs apart, place a rope* (a belt or tie will also work) around your thighs at the knees. Clench out against the rope and hold for five seconds at least and release. Do this as many times as you can. Twenty or more reps and you should feel it.

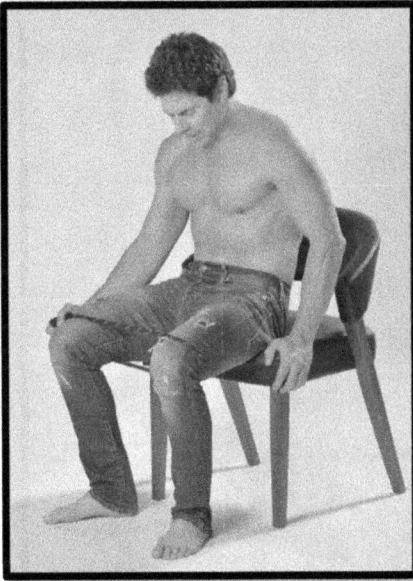

Instead of using an applied restraint, if you have a desk with sides close to your legs you can try pushing out with your thighs. Just be sure to apply force evenly unless the desk is otherwise secured from moving.

(see also LEVEL III: #1 BUTT and LEG EXERCISES – g) Sitting Hip Abductor for a version using an elastic band.)

HINT: for an extra burn, keep your butt raised off the seat (it's also a good idea for life).

NOTE: #9 THE THIGHS – d) Sitting Hip Adductor is a good companion exercise. It also works the glutes.

#2 THE STOMACH (Abdominals or Abs)

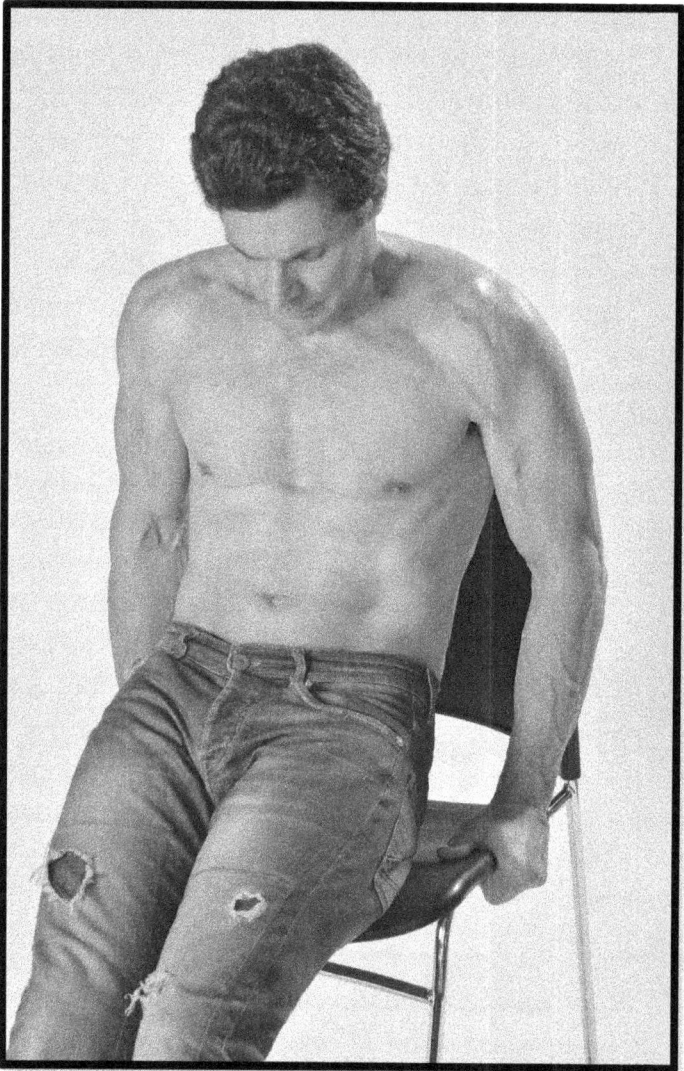

The abs are another big muscle group that you basically can't overwork. But do try as often as you remember. Billy obviously remembers a lot.

This is a muscle group that can be exercised almost anywhere. A perfect, unused task time to clench your abs is while sitting or lying around watching television, especially when slouching on a chair or on a couch. In this position it's very easy to isolate the front and the sides (the obliques) of your stomach. Also, the time while walking or just standing and waiting is greatly under-used. And although, while driving is a little harder to engage the stomach muscles, you still can. Watching TV, walking and driving are all empty, time-slot gold mines.

Clenching your abs can be done with or without moving your torso and while standing, sitting, lying down, running or walking. And until it becomes habit, it bears repeating that these exercises can be done – and should be done – as often as you remember and are able, especially the non-moving Isometric version, depending, of course, on where you are and what you're doing.

HINT: Sucking your stomach in will enhance the burn and if you are trying to impress someone around you, it looks better anyway.

WARNING: Stomach Clench Crunches should be conducted with caution while driving (just as should doing any exercise be, when your attention is needed elsewhere). This is absolutely not the time to visualize anything other than the goal ahead of you, like the road. So, engage carefully.

a) <u>Stomach Clench and Stomach Clench Crunch</u>

Standing: Clench an area of your abs as hard as you can. With a slight shift of your torso and a little concentration, you can isolate and fully engage your upper or lower abs or your sides (the obliques). However, clenching your sides might also engage your lats, but to a lesser extent. Do what feels best for you.

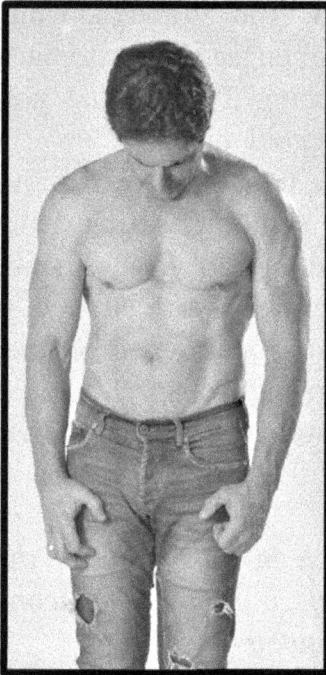

Sitting: Hold your legs up* as you clench. It adds to the burn plus works your thighs.

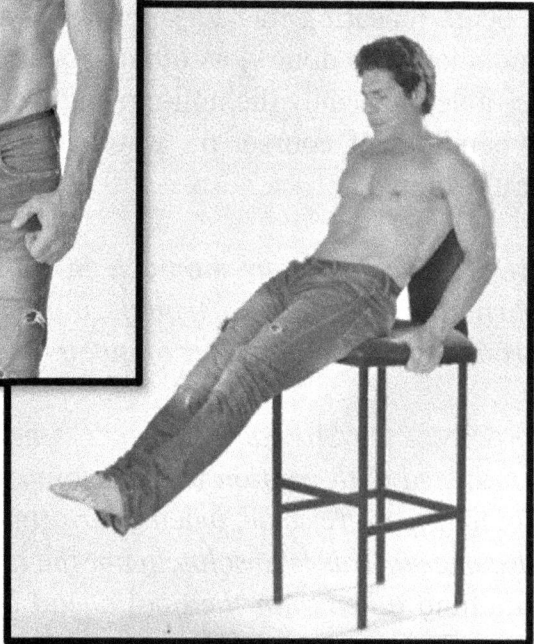

*bring your knees up to your chest, and hold for an extra crunch.

Lying down: With your legs on the floor, raise your upper body, clench and hold. Lower and do it again.

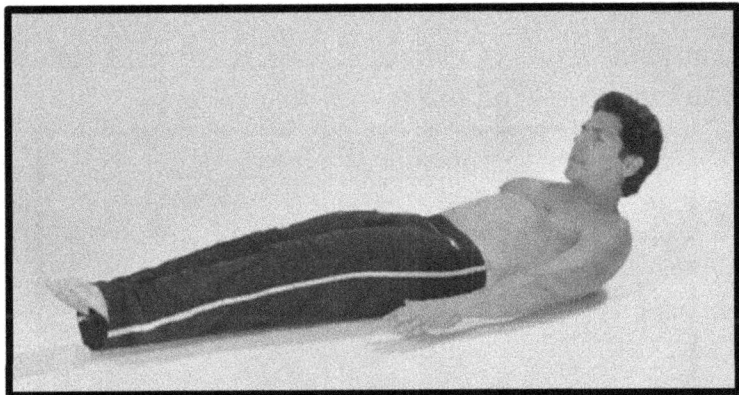

Lying down (with a leg lift): Start by lying flat, raise your legs and upper body, clench your abs, HOLD and release. Then do it again.

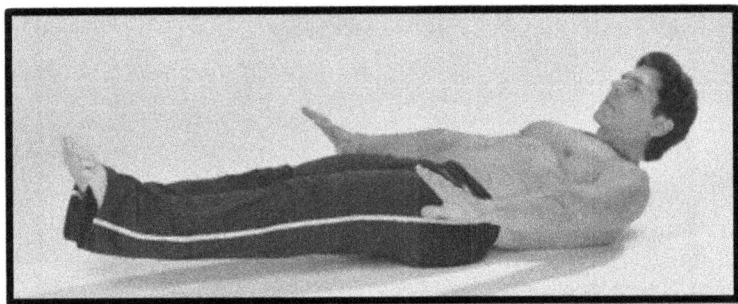

Whether you're doing a Clench or Clench Crunch, try to hold and tighten your abs for at least a ten count and then do it again until you really, really feel it.

NOTE: *When either standing, sitting or lying down, your clenches can be intensified by* <u>crunching</u> *your neck and torso closer to the area you're engaging.*

#3 THE BICEPS

With the following exercises, you'll find that when you really work your biceps, your pecs might also be worked as well and sometimes your triceps.

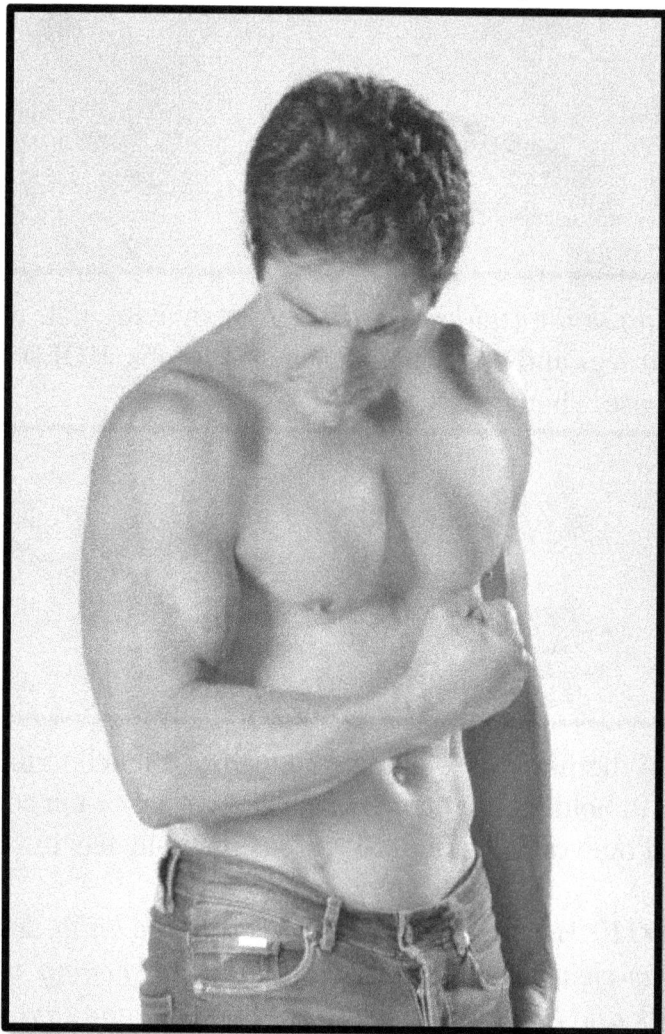

a) <u>Curl Clench Pump</u> (no resistance)

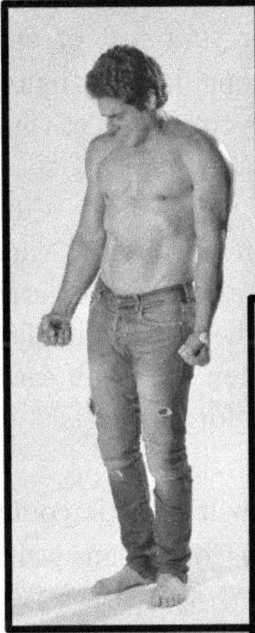

Grip some imaginary weights with both hands* extended down at your thighs. Now tighten your fists, clenching your biceps hard as you pump the "weights" up to your chest (one to four seconds per pump-up is good). Exhale at the top of the move and inhale as you release your muscles going down.

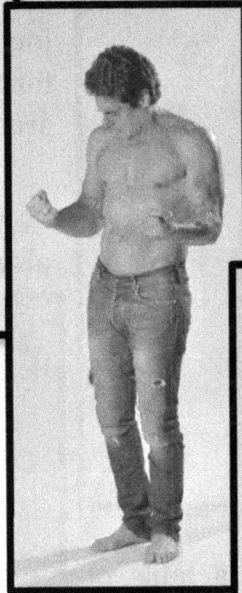

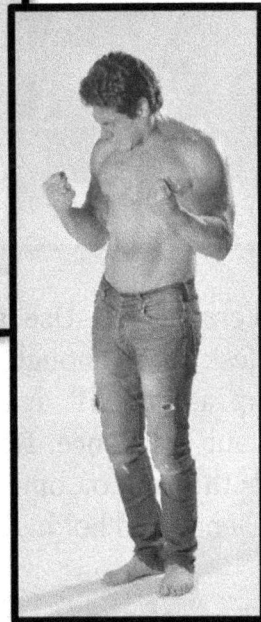

Do three sets of ten to twenty reps, even if you spread them out over the day.

Alternate Version: Clench your biceps for at least three to five seconds for each of the three stationary positions shown. Do as many reps as you can.

*or use just one arm at a time.

b) <u>Stationary Curl Clench</u>

Version #1: Secure a rope* under your feet or any immovable object. Griping the rope in one hand, clench your bicep as you try to pull your fist up to your shoulders.

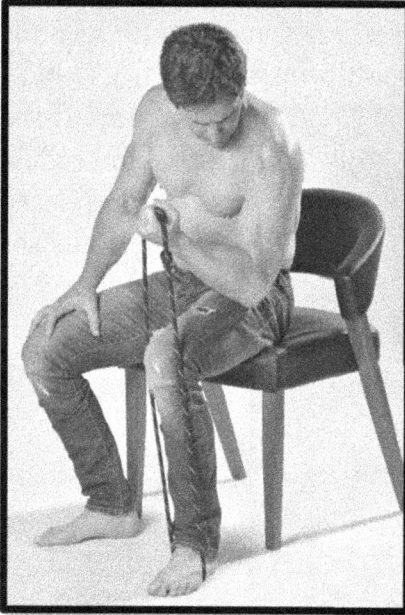

Like the Curl Clench Pump, vary the angle of your arm for better results. Try for ten reps with each arm for three sets.

*a belt or a tie could also work just as well.

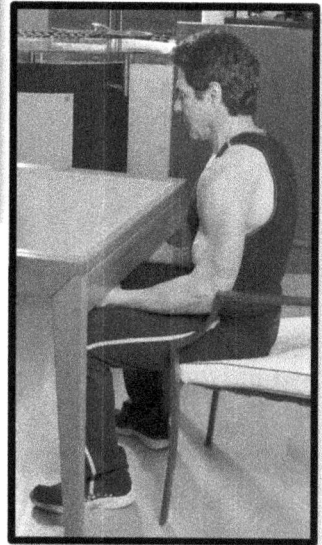

Version #2: Use a table or desk heavy enough to not rise up as you lift against it for your resistance. Do this with both arms or one at a time. Clench and hold.

WARNING: DO NOT try this while driving.

#4 THE CHEST (Pectorals or Pecs)

The chest muscles, as a group, are hard to isolate, though we're sure you know where to look. Exercising them often engages the triceps, lats, shoulders and sometimes biceps. But don't let that stop you. Unfortunately, the pecs are also hard muscles to get a vigorous workout for in STAGE 1 (LEVEL I) and STAGE 2. Hard, but not impossible.

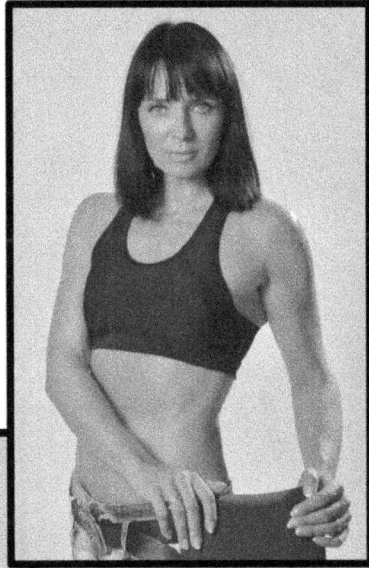

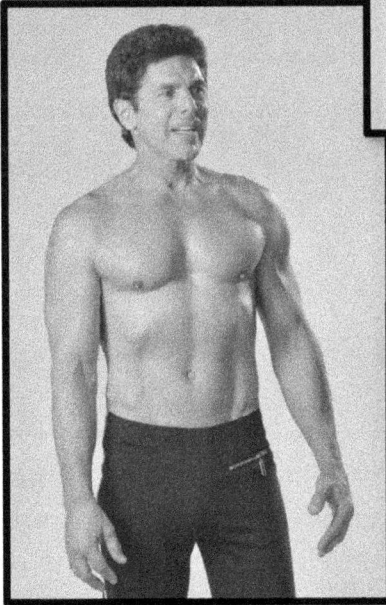

NOTE: Although there isn't a chest exercise much better than old-fashioned push-ups, they generally go far beyond isometrics or beginning exercises, however, an Angled Push-Up Chest Clench is included later in this section.

a) <u>Stationary Chest Clench</u>*

Version #1: Place your cupped hands against your thighs, with fingers spread. Press in, arch your back and clench your pecs hard as you can. Hold for at least a five-count, release and repeat for as many reps as you're able.

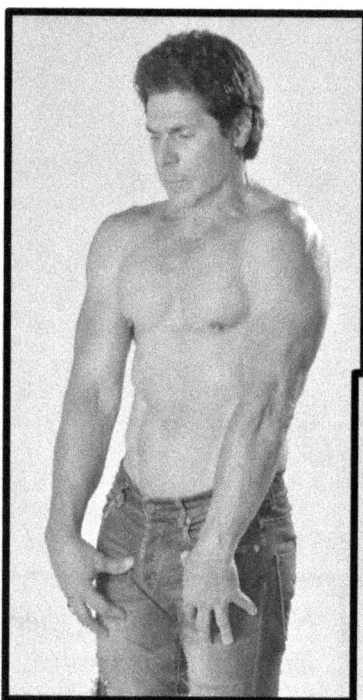

<u>This one is also great for the abs.</u>

*below picture taken 2017

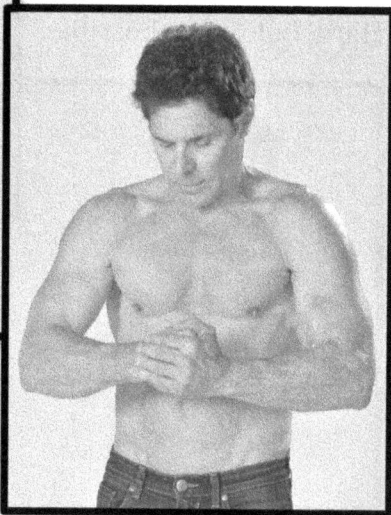

Version #2: With hands together at your chest (fist into open palm) press them against each other as you clench your pecs hard, with equal force. Adjust your form until you've isolated your chest as best you can. Try holding the clench for a ten count or longer and do enough reps to really feel it.

b) <u>Leaning Chest Clench</u>

Leaning with your hands on a wall (desk; counter; anything that won't move), place your feet together or apart (your choice) and as far away from the resisting object as you feel comfortable. Place your hands apart, past your shoulders and keeping your back straight, clench your pecs and hold for a ten count. Do as many reps as you can, making sure to rest between them by standing upright.

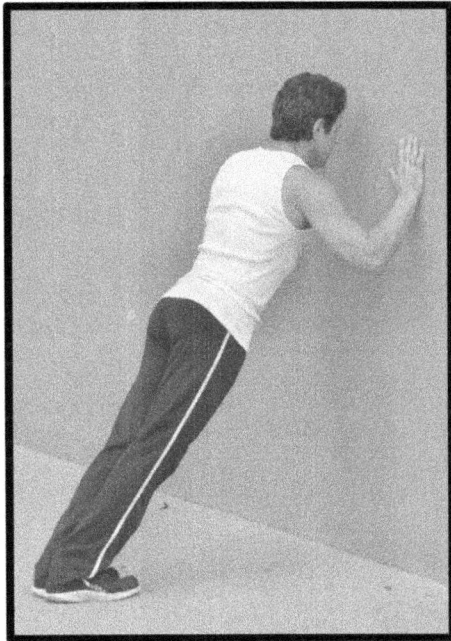

BONUS: Try also clenching your lats, hamstrings, thighs, glutes, triceps or abs. You might as well get the most out of things that you can. So, clench them all!

WARNING: Make sure your feet are planted securely so your legs won't slip out from under you.

(see also **LEVEL II**: #3 PUSH-UPS – b) Angled Push-Ups, for a moving version.)

c) <u>Casual Chest Clench</u>

Yes, Billy is "performing" an exercise, though his posing isn't necessary. Try the following:

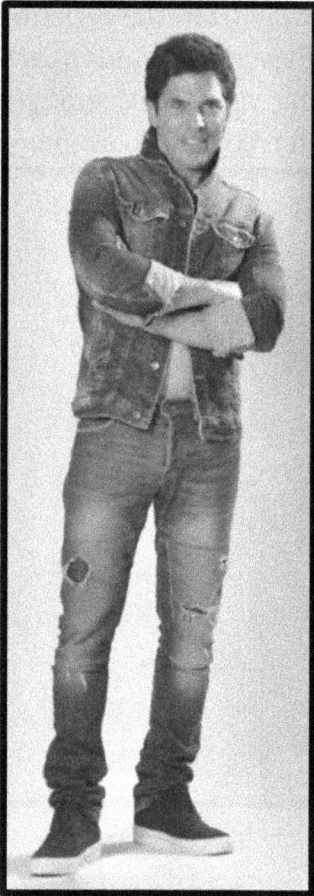

Without resistance (shown) – cross your arms over your chest, clenching your pecs as hard as you can. Hold for about a three count and release for as many reps as you feel able. You can also work only one pec at a time, just work each side equally.

With resistance (not shown) – place one hand or fist under the other elbow and press up, clenching the pec on that side. Switch elbows and repeat as above.

With practice, these exercises will look like you're simply crossing your arms, unless you're showing too much strain. In fact, if you're showing excessive strain on your face during this or any exercise, then stop it. Your face muscles aren't the ones you should be engaging, unless your smiling. But how strange or silly you look is up to you... and Billy.

#5 THE UPPER BACK (Latissimus Dorsi or Lats)

The back is a large group of muscles, so try to do exercises that engage them as often as you can. We are concentrating here on the area at the outer edges of your upper back that extends from your armpits and angles down and in, almost to your waist.

During STAGE 1 – LEVEL I, it will be almost impossible to work your lats enough. But try anyway.

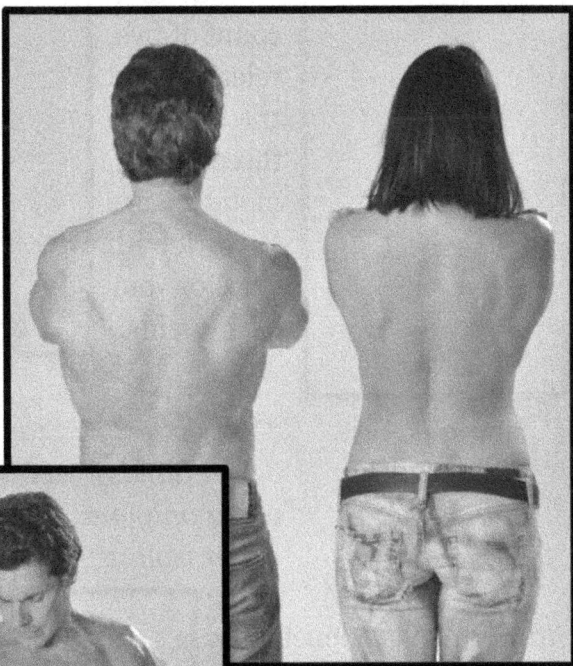

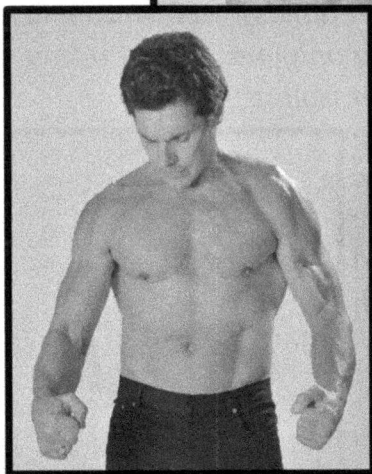

Sorry. This may not be the front view you were hoping to see, but it does show off Billy's clenched lats pretty well.

a) <u>Stationary Lats Clench</u>*

Standing: With either an open hand or closed fist, press against your thigh(s), clenching your lats hard on that side (or sides)**.

(with open hands)

(with closed fist)

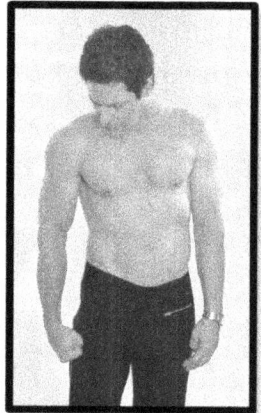

Hold for a count of five, release and try to do three sets, making sure to work both sides of your back evenly.

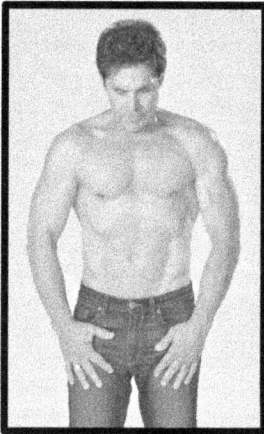

*above picture taken 2017

***Except for Standing (with open hands), we recommend using only one arm at a time to better isolate your lats.*

*Sitting: A*s you clench your lats it will also work the shoulders, chest and stomach. Do as above with one arm, then the other.

Suggestion: In public, you might want a shirt.

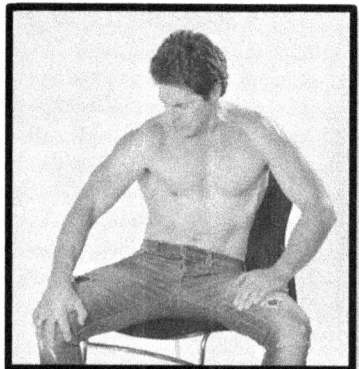

b) <u>Lats Lift Clench</u>

While sitting in a chair with sturdy armrests, grip the arms, rise up slightly and clench your lats hard. This will also work your triceps. You don't have to raise yourself high up for this, but you can. In fact try experimenting at varying intervals to see which position gives you the best workout. You can also try resting your forearms on the armrests and simply raising up just enough to clench your lats.

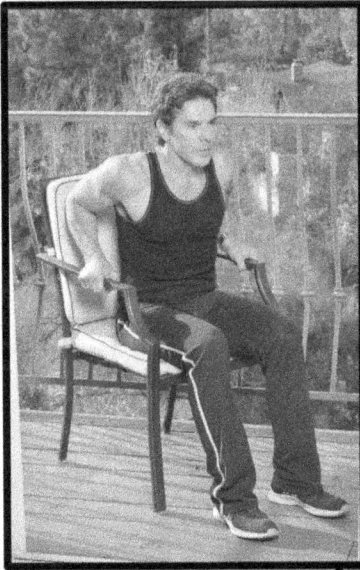

Hold the clench for a five to ten count for ten reps or until you are really able to feel it – or whenever you find yourself sitting around.

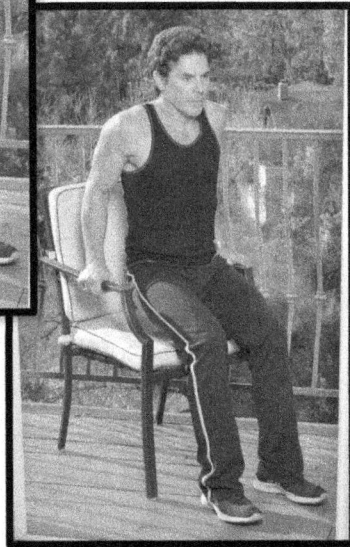

NOTE: *For a moving version, see LEVEL II: #4 CURLS, LIFTS and PUSHES – i) Moving Lats Lift)*

#6 THE NECK

The neck is often an overlooked muscle group. And chances are you're overlooking it right now.

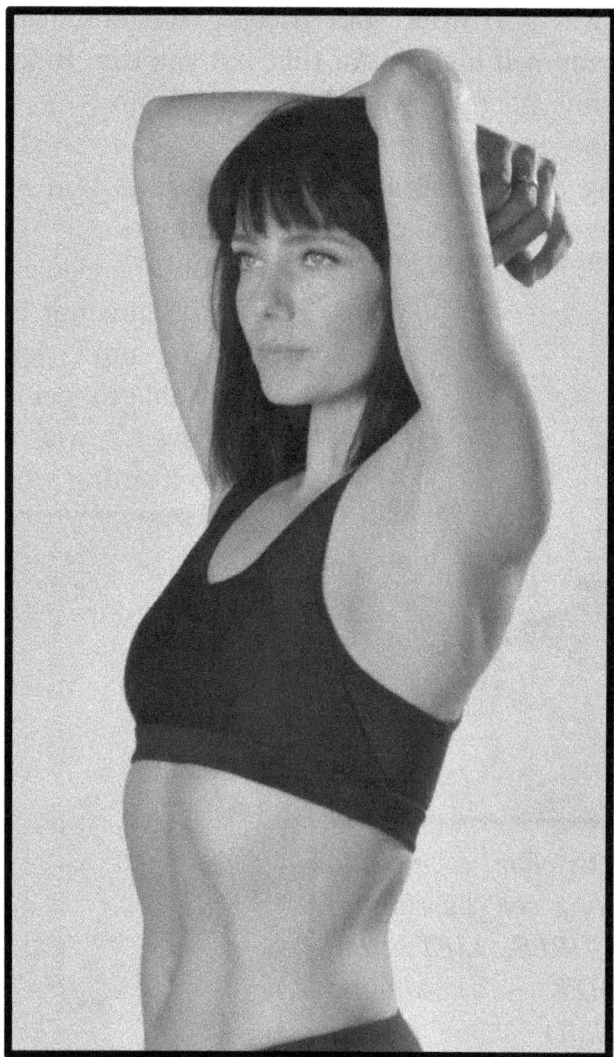

a) <u>Neck Push Clench</u>

While standing, clasp your hands behind your head. Push forward with your hands as you resist with your head for a stationary neck clench. Hold for at least a three-count, for ten reps.

Now with your neck turned slightly to one side, push and resist, clenching your neck for ten reps. Turn your head to the other side for ten more reps.

Finally, place both hands over your forehead and push and resist for one last stationary clench for ten reps.

Do three sets total for all four positions.

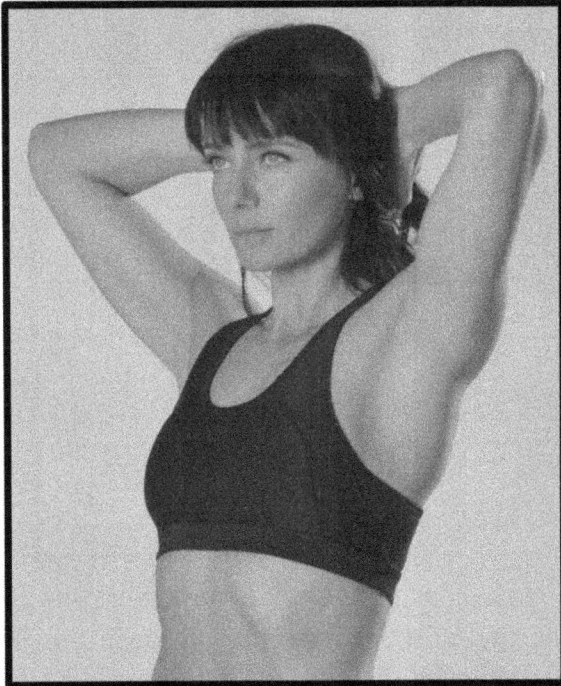

Clench but DON'T STRAIN!

This is an important clench, especially for those working at the computer or sitting at a desk for long stretches.

#7 THE TRICEPS

We can pretty much guess you are again looking in the wrong place. The triceps are the muscles that run along the back of the arms from the elbows to the shoulders.

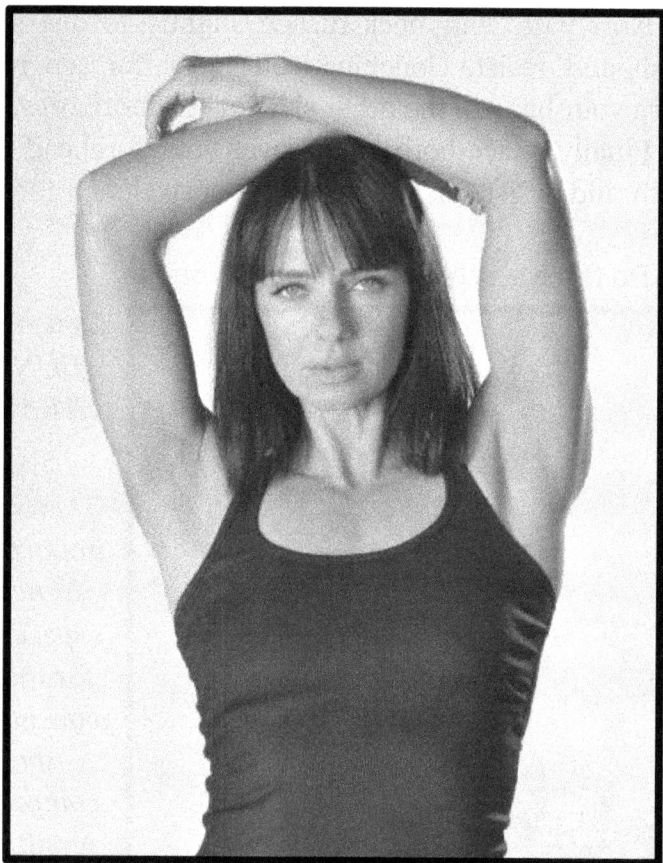

Although push-ups are one of the best exercises for many muscles including the triceps, following are a couple good substitutes.

a) <u>Stationary Triceps Clench</u>*

Straighten one arm at a time and bring it backwards as far as you can while clenching that arm's triceps. As you hold the clench for at least a five count try clenching even harder and moving your arm back even farther. After at least three reps, do the same move with your other arm. Do as many sets as comfortable.

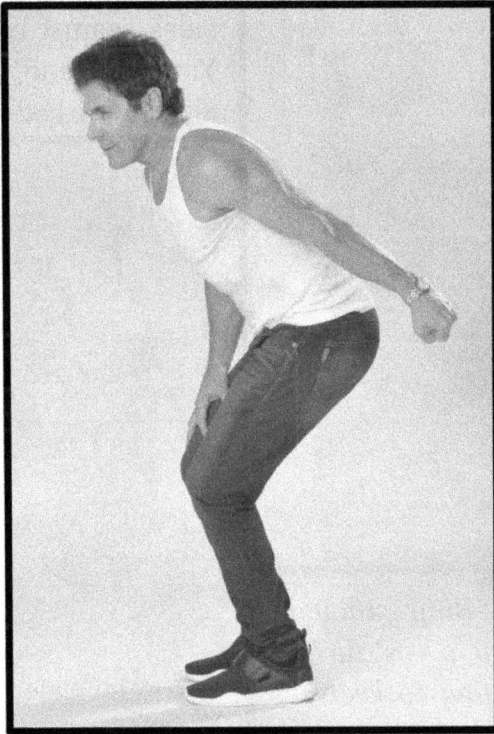

*picture taken 2017

NOTE: *By bending at the waist as Billy is doing, a secondary clench in your supporting arm can be achieved, though to a much lesser extent.*

b) <u>Triceps Pull/Push Clench</u>*

Pulling: Using a twisted-up hand towel or similar cloth, firmly grasp the towel at both ends and pull each arm against the other, trying to isolate your triceps. This will also work your lats to some extent.

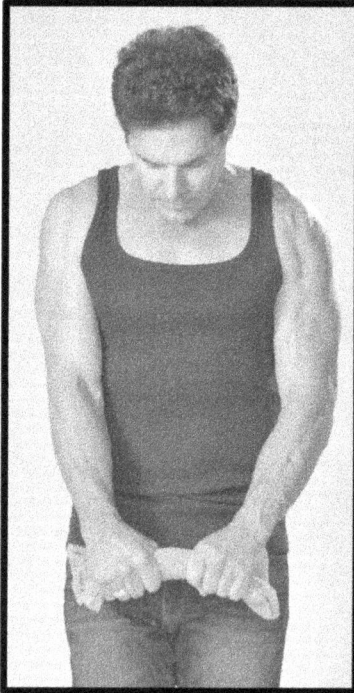

Pushing: Using the same aid, cross one wrist over the other and push to the sides against each other. Your lats and chest will also be worked.

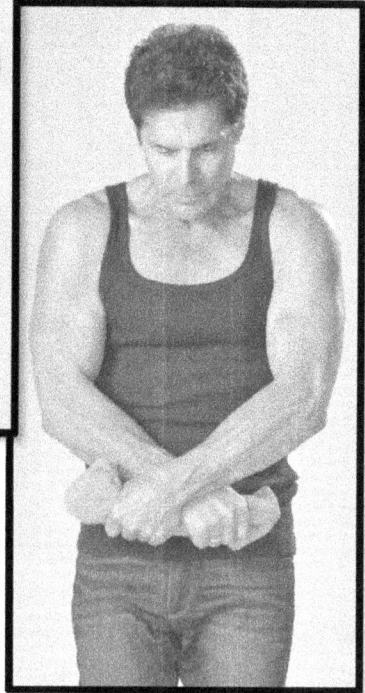

NOTE: *Billy thought this up at a restaurant, while trying to keep his temper over someone eating with their mouth open. So clench hard!*

*pictures taken 2017

c) Triceps Push-Back Clench

This exercise is best performed against a wall (or some other shoulder-high immovable object). With your feet together, stand about two or three feet away from the wall and lean all the way forward against your forearms. Raise your elbows away from the wall, pushing in with the sides of your fists until you are able to isolate and engage your triceps. Clench hard and hold it for a   ten-count.   Do three sets of ten reps.

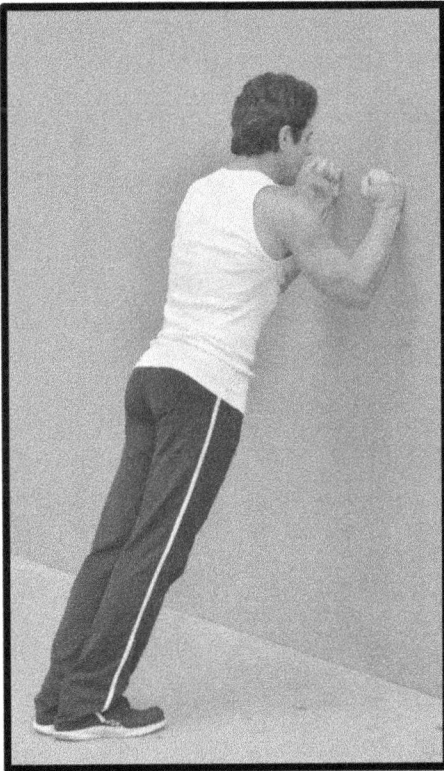

BONUS: Clench your butt and abs for   some   extra burns.

ALTERNATIVES: *Any clench for the triceps that uses an immovable   object for resistance will also work. (i.e. while sitting, press out with the back of one wrist against your inner thigh, clenching that arm's triceps – use caution if performed while driving).*

#8 THE FOREARMS ("The Popeye Muscle")

The forearms are often neglected muscles that affect your wrist strength and overall appearance.

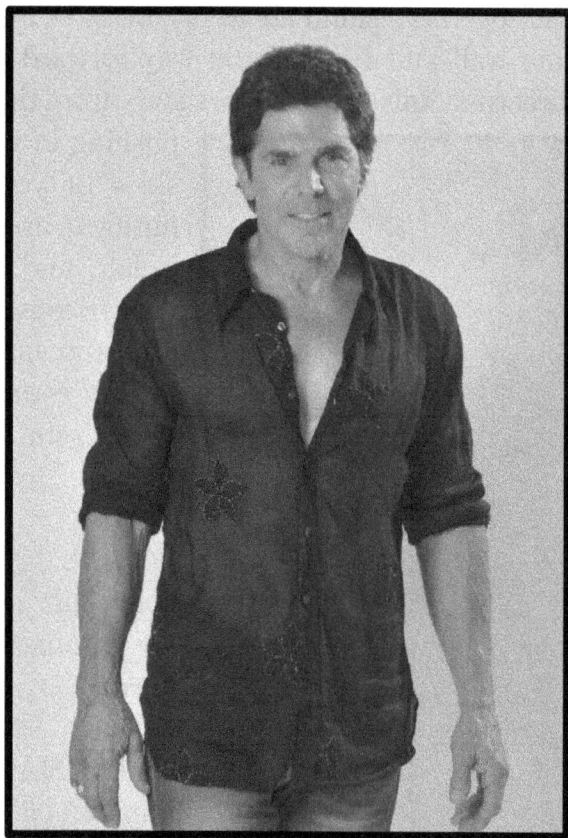

NOTE: *Unlike Popeye, spinach won't directly help you with this or any muscle. And though a spinach salad can be great, be sure to check your teeth when finished. "I wrongly assumed a good friend (Tim) would tell me a front tooth was greened out." – Billy*

a) <u>Freestyle Forearm Clench</u>

VERSION #1: Simply extend your arm down to your side, make a tight fist and bend your wrist toward you, engaging your forearm for a good, long clench. Do the same thing by bending your wrist away from you. Work both forearms evenly, until you feel them burning. Clenching your forearms in this manner will work the muscles on both the top and bottom of your wrists.

VERSION #2: Clench your forearms as you very slowly move your wrists up and down, increasing the effectiveness of the clench. Again, do this until you feel it.

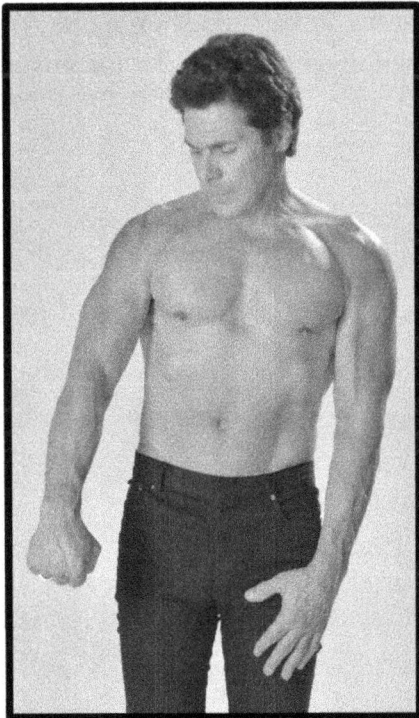

NOTE: *These clenches can be done quite easily without drawing much attention to what you're doing unless, like Billy, you insist on exercising your ego along with your forearms... shirtless.*

b) Side Forearm Clench

This exercise is similar to #5 THE UPPER BACK – a) Stationary Lats Clench (with closed fist), except that this time the wrist is turned to the side and pressed against the thigh. Try not to engage any muscle other than the forearm. Hold for a ten-count, release and clench again for at least ten reps. Do the same with the other wrist. Try performing more sets whenever you think of it, throughout the day.

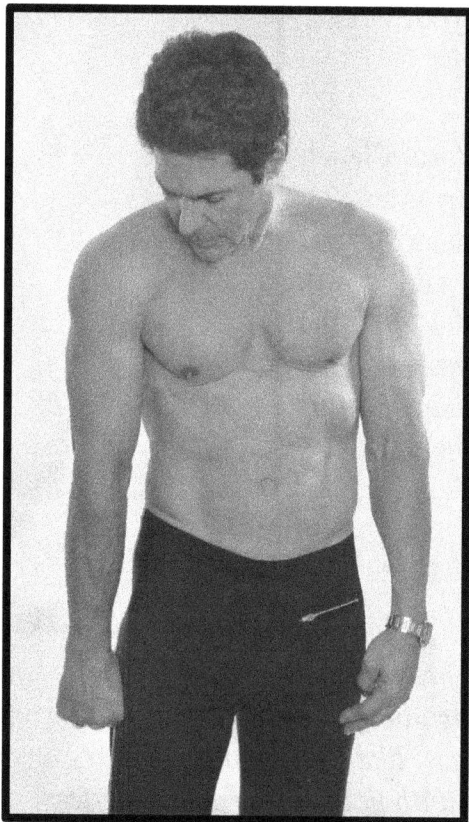

#9 THE THIGHS (Quadriceps or Quads)

Thighs are the kind of muscles that, when exerting an opposite force against them, are often fairly difficult to totally isolate during a clench. And the more you can isolate a muscle, the better the results.

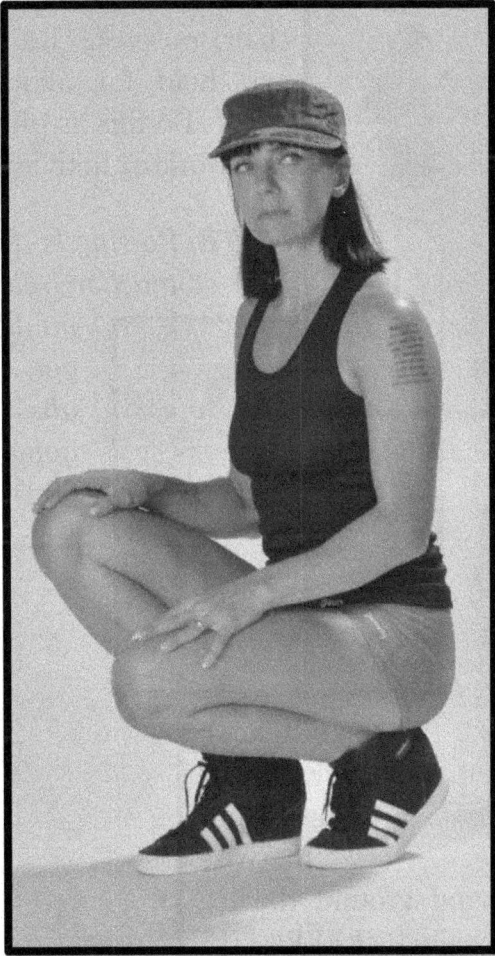

a) Sitting Upper-Leg Clench

This exercise isolates your thighs the best with a good hard clench, especially when working one leg at a time. It also strengthens your hips.

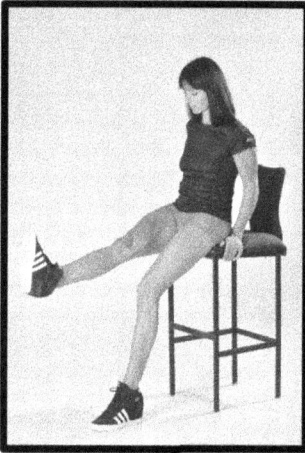

Version #1: While sitting on a chair, raise one leg (or both) and hold for about a ten-count. Do this as often as you can, working both legs evenly.

NOTE: *Raising both legs also uses stomach muscles, so you might as well get a good abs clench going while you're at it.*

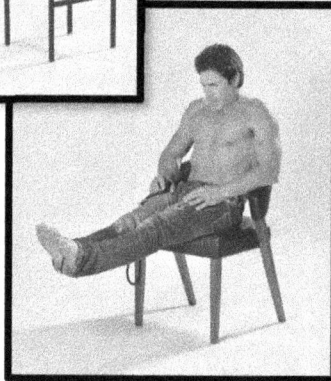

Again, Billy just likes taking off his shirt.

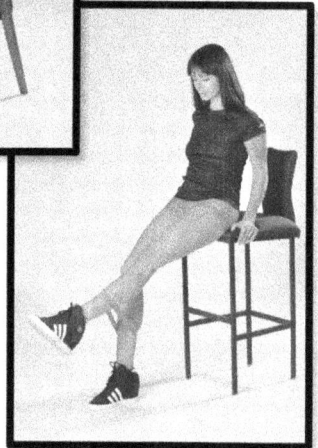

Version #2 (with resistance): Use a belt, band or similar object hooked under your other leg (or otherwise secured) and around the leg being clenched. KEEP THE CLENCHED LEG STARIGHT.

b) Lying-Down Upper-Leg Clench

This exercise is performed by clenching only one thigh at a time. Clenching both thighs at once tends to decrease the effectiveness of the clench and, if raising both legs will mainly engage your abs.

Version #1: While lying on your back, on a soft surface, with legs flat on the floor, tense and clench the thigh of one leg. You should be able to really lock it in. Hold the clench for at least a five-count, release and repeat for at least five reps – more if you can.

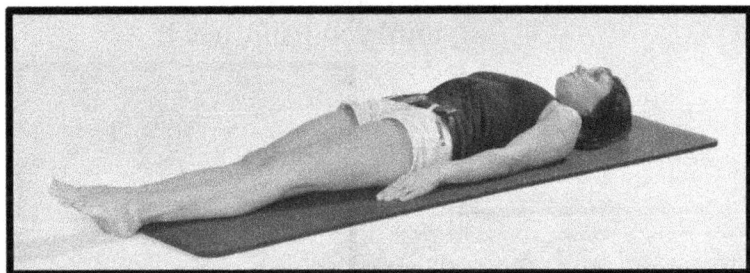

Version #2: Do this the same as Version #1 only this time raise the leg slightly that's being clenched. Raising the leg is harder, but gives a stronger burn.

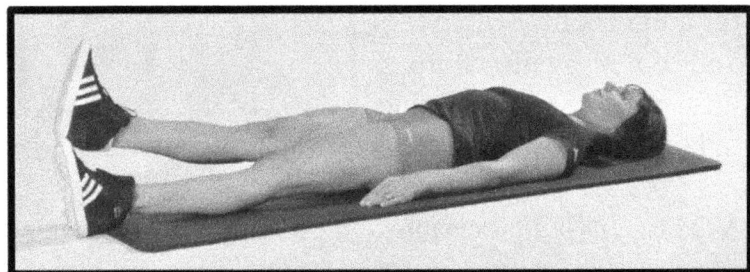

NOTE: *Style changes aren't required – that's Inara.*

c) Pushing Upper-Leg Clench

This exercise works the quads and the hamstrings almost equally, however, it works them on opposite legs, but mostly it's great for the Hip Flexors.

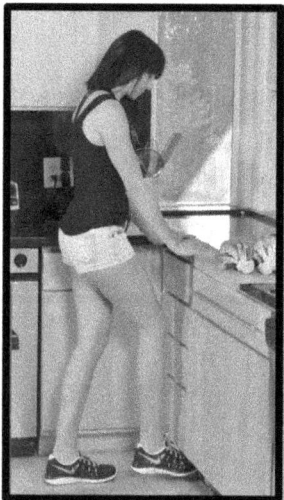

Version #1: While standing in front of an immovable object such as a counter or sofa, push against it with one leg as you push back with the other, for a ten-count. Do the same with your other leg. And keep it up it until you really feel it.

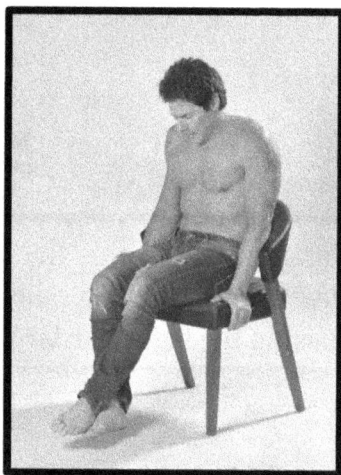

Version #2: Cross your legs at the ankles and pull in with the top leg while pushing out with the other for a ten count. Switch legs and do it again. With a little practice you'll be able to fatigue your thighs and hamstrings pretty well.

NOTE: *In both versions, if pushing forward with your right leg you will also feel it burn on the hamstring of your left leg and vice-versa.*

d) <u>Sitting Hip Adductor Clench</u>

Though this is actually more of a workout for the inner thighs, it's also a good one for the overall shape of the butt* and another great one for the office.

For this exercise to be the most effective, you'll need an object to place between your knees for variable resistance, such as a rolled up sweater or towel or even a paperback book. While sitting, with your choice of resistance held between your knees, press your legs together as hard as you can.

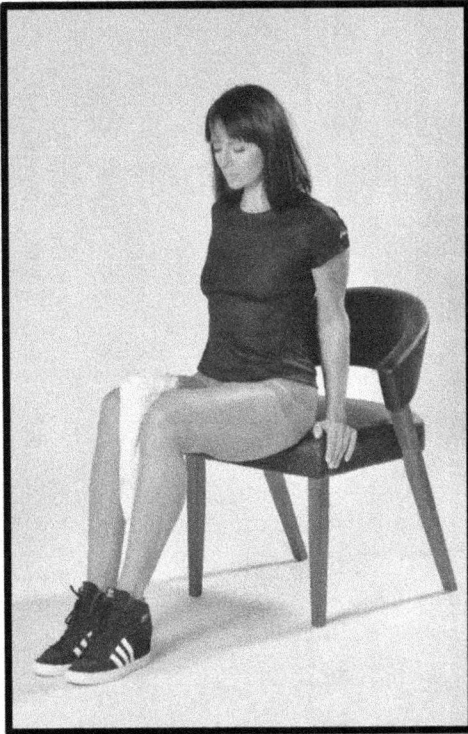

You may have to experiment a little to feel it effectively in your glutes because your inner thighs are worked the easiest. Just keep clenching until you do and you've had enough.

NOTE: #1 THE BUTT – g) Sitting Hip Abductor Clench is a great companion move.

*again, raising off your butt gives a better glute burn.

#10 THE CALVES

The calves are often overlooked muscles that are usually attractive when developed. You don't need huge calves, but a little bit of definition is always nice.

No, we're sorry. Those aren't calves.

Nope. Not there either. But you're getting warmer. Just a little further down.

There you go. Right between the knee and the ankle.

Okay. Now you can go back up and take in the whole picture. We told you calves are nice to look at.

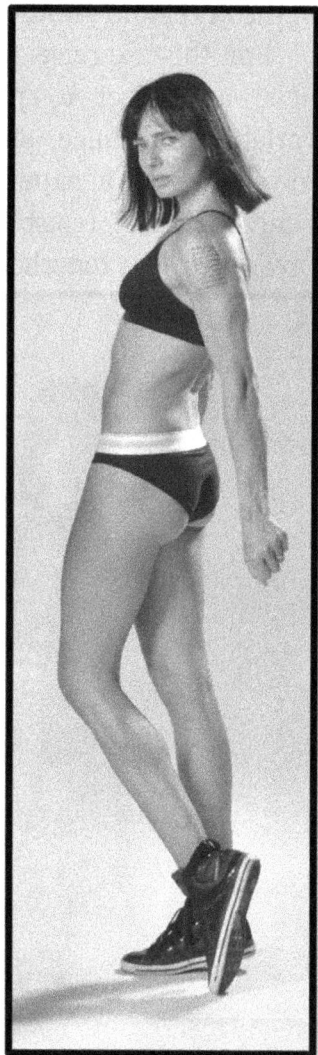

a) <u>Rising Calf Clench</u>

While holding the back of a chair for balance – or a desk, counter or anything sturdy, that's about waist high – rise up on the toes of one foot, trying not to use any other muscle, but your calf. Clench that calf for a three-count and come back down. About ten reps per calf is good, making sure to rest between sets.

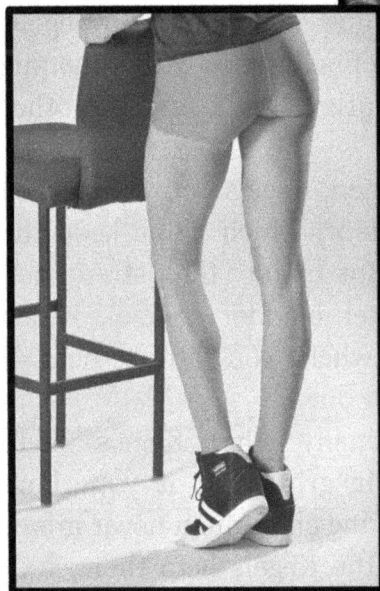

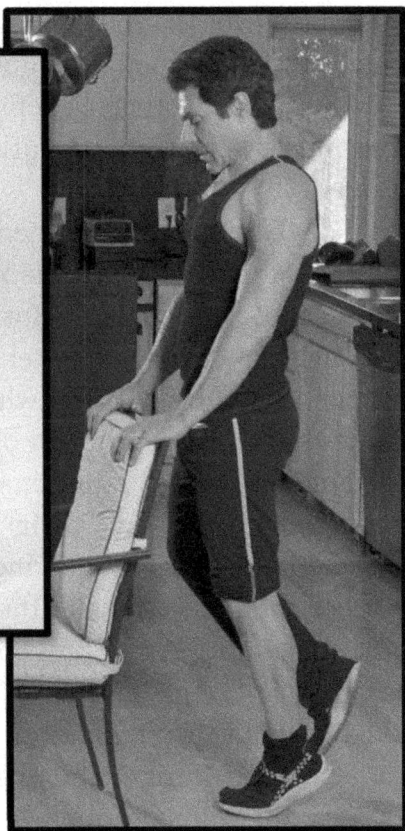

NOTE: *You can try rising up with both calves at once, but it's not quite as effective.*

WARNING: Be careful. Calves can cramp easily.

#11 THE KEGELS (The Private Place)

Not everyone has heard of these, but everyone does them in one form or another, generally without thinking about it. You use them most when in the bathroom or when waiting to go and trying not to. In other words, during the process of elimination. To be precise, Kegels are actually the name of the man who discovered the exercises and not the muscles. But for our purposes they will be synonymous. Kegels, however, have other benefits besides strengthening the muscles that control urine flow... and the other thing.

For both women and men, Kegels help strengthen what's called the pelvic floor, which helps keep the pelvic muscles in place. But mainly they strengthen the urinary tract for better bladder control, which comes in quite handy when you aren't near a bathroom or are waiting for one.

For women, additionally the Kegels help strengthen, let's say, their grip. And if you don't understand what we're talking about then never mind.

For men, additionally the Kegels help them, let's say, make a firmer impression for a longer period of time. And again, if you can't figure out what we're talking about then move on.

The good thing about these exercises is that you can do them almost anywhere in pretty much total privacy. And they work.

a) <u>Kegel Clench</u>

If you aren't sure how to engage your Kegel exercise muscles, an easy way to tell that you are doing them right is, the next time you are using the bathroom, stop your flow of urine. Those are your Kegel exercise muscles. Now that you know what they feel like when you use them, try this exercise. Standing or sitting, it doesn't matter.

Do a Kegel Clench hard and hold it for about five seconds and release. Just make sure you aren't engaging any other muscle at the same time. Repeat this clench again and again for about one or two commercial breaks. You may or may not see any physical changes, per say, but over time you should feel the effects. So, keep clenching. It's good for you.

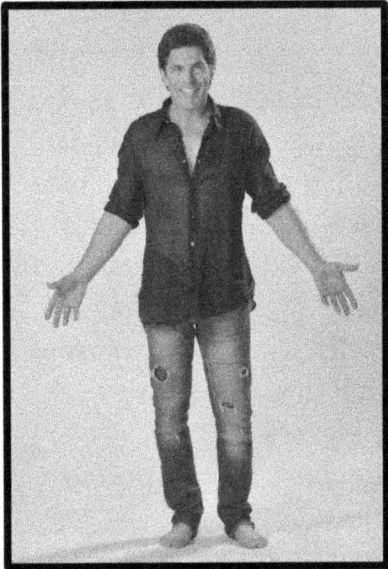

Who knows if Billy is really doing a Kegel here or not.

After all, it's a hands-free move, so he could be.

Maybe that's why he's smiling.

#12 DUO CLENCHES

This section includes clenches that can be done with a partner. Some are stationary and some involve movement. They all involve cooperation.

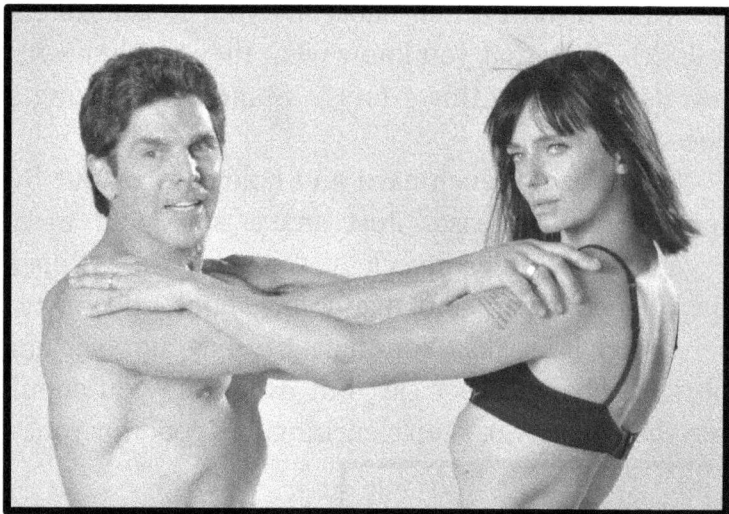

For example, in the picture above, Billy is feebly trying to pull Inara toward him and Inara is calmly pushing Billy away (or possibly readying her hands to clench his neck); an exercise that Billy is used to.

But seriously, one of the extra benefits of duo exercises is that, generally, while one person is working one set of muscles the other person is working a different set of muscles.

NOTE: *What Billy is doing above is not working*.*

**WARNING: Serious injury (to Billy) could result.*

a) <u>Duo Sitting Abs/Chest Press Clench</u>

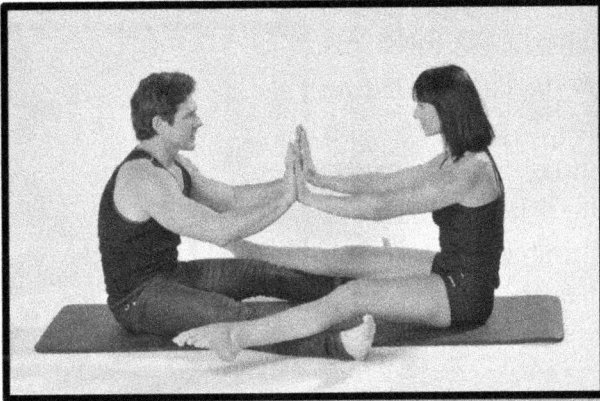

Face each other with overlapping outstretched legs and press your palms against each other, clenching your abs and chest. Do this until one of you gives up.

b) <u>Duo Standing Abs/Chest/Thighs/Butt Clench</u>

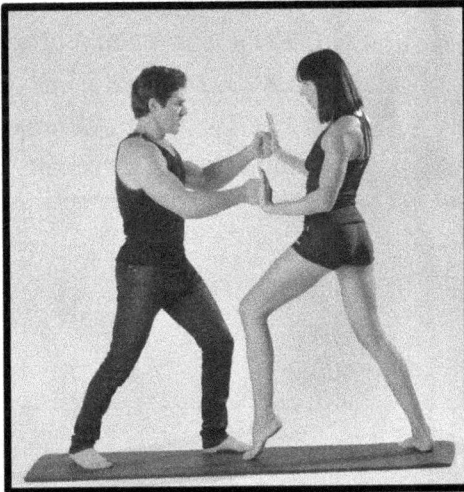

Face each other with legs wide, one in front of the other. One person pushes as the other resists with their fists into each other's open palms, with each clenching their abs and chest. Steady yourselves by clenching your thighs and butt. Switch back and forth (with fists and palms) until tired.

c) Duo Standing Chest/Triceps Press Clench

Facing – forearms against forearms – one person pushes in (clenching their chest) and the other pushes out (clenching their triceps). Switch arm positions for about five to ten reps.

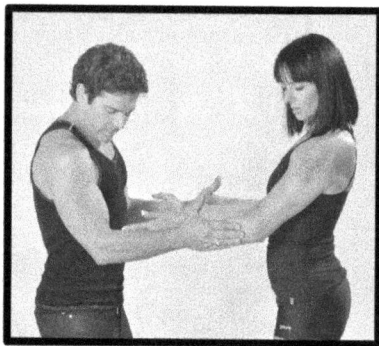

d) Duo Standing Biceps/Chest Press Clench

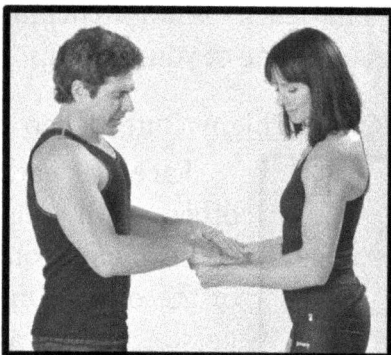

Facing each other, one person pushes down with their open hands (clenching their chest), as the other pushes up with their fists turned sideways (clenching their biceps).

Do equally, for each person, for about five to ten reps.

SUGGESTION: Try varying the height of your hands or adding movement through the clench.

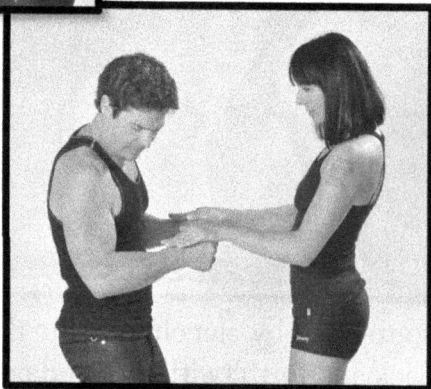

e) Duo Upper Leg/Abs Clench

While lying down, clench your quads and abs (and your butt) in stages as below, as your partner resists. Increase and decrease the resistance or try raising one leg at a time to alter your workout. These won't be easy but they're effective.

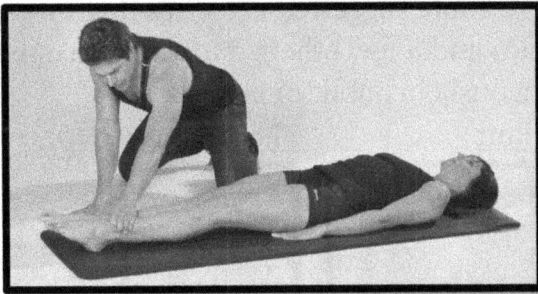

(see also LEVEL III: #8 DUO EXERCISES – b) Duo Upper Leg Lifts)

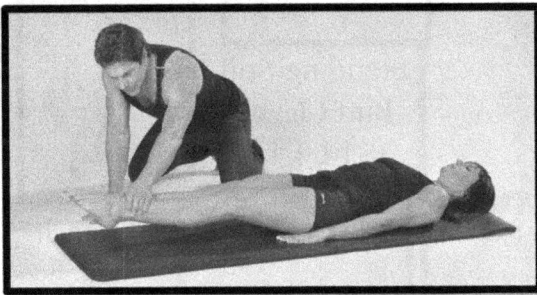

After you've done as many as you can, switch positions with your partner.

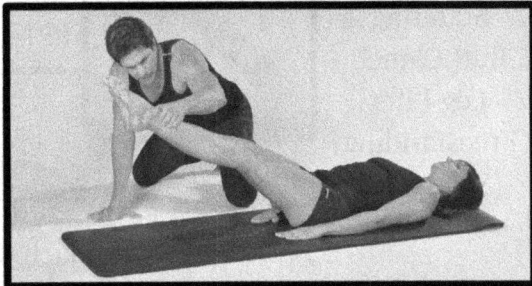

Daily/Weekly Exercise Suggestions (LEVEL I)

If you aren't able to do a series of **Xer-tasks** each day or several times during the week, then try to do at least one that, with a little persistence, will become a daily habit. And once one becomes a habit, it will be much easier to make further exercising a habit, too.

Following are some suggested exercises that target the main muscles and a few others. Most can be done fairly inconspicuously in public or at work.

The Butt   The Stomach

Standing-Still
Butt Clench
(S1-L I-1a)

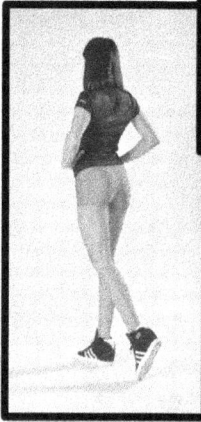

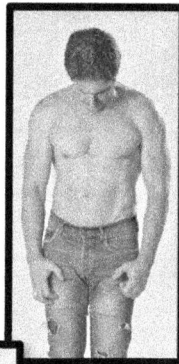

Standing
Butt Clench
Leg Lifts
(Freestanding)
(S1-L I-1d)

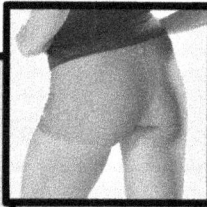

Stomach
Clench
(Sitting)
(S1-L I-2a)

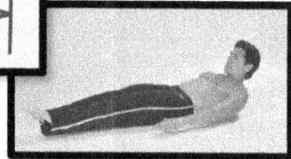

Stomach
Clench
(Standing)
(S1-L I-2a)

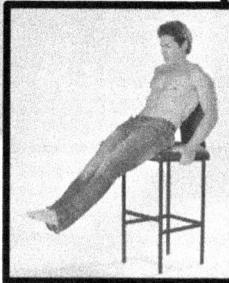

Stomach Clench Crunch
(Lying Down) (S1-L I-2a)

The Kegels

The Upper Back

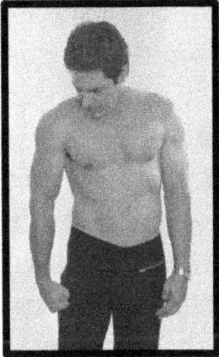

The Biceps

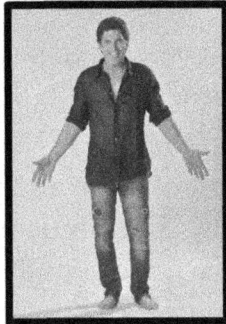

Kegel Clench
(S1-L I-11a)

Stationary
Lats Clench
(closed fist)
(S1-L I-5a)

The Neck

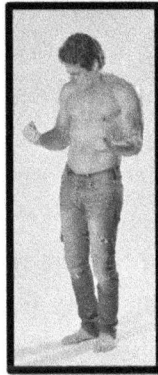

Curl Clench
Pump
(S1-L I-3a)

The Chest

The Triceps

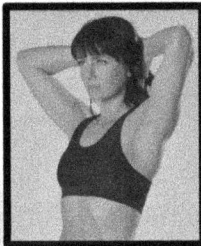

Neck Push
Clench
(S1-L I-6a)

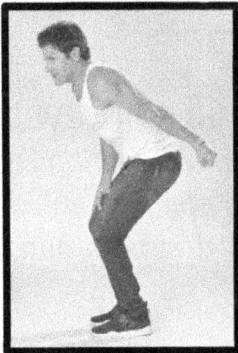

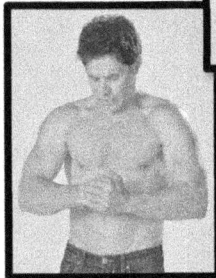

Stationary
Triceps Clench
(S1-L I-7a)

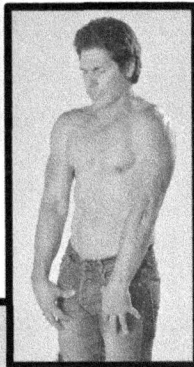

Stationary
Chest
Clench
(Version #1)
(S1-L I-4a)

Stationary Chest Clench (Version #2) (S1-L I-4a)

LEVEL II: Muscle Movement

This section involves mainly isokinetic exercises rather than isometric. And unless you're watching television or doing some other activity that doesn't require the majority of your attention, a bit of time management might be needed. So, check your schedule. We're sure you can find a few moments that are basically wasted on a task that doesn't need them. (i.e. during commercials; waiting for the bathroom to be free; reading a gossip magazine for the third time).

Most of these exercises should be familiar to you, though doing them may not. And that's the only trick – doing them. Remember, it's not necessary to perform more than one exercise in a session. If you have the time, great. But STAGE 1 only requires that you find the time to share or spare for an Xer-task, not how many you actually do or how often.

Hint: When doing any of the exercises in LEVEL II (and LEVEL III) try to remember what clenching each muscle felt like in LEVEL I. This should help you engage, visualize and increase your desired results.

Suggested Accessories*:
    Exercise mat, Yoga mat or rug
    Medicine-Ball
    Elastic band

*again, do the exercises of your choice, your way.

#1 BUTT and BACK LEG EXERCISES

While Squats and Lunges target the butt they also engage the quads (especially just above the knees) and, depending on your feet position, the inner thighs. Upper Back Leg Lifts basically work the butt, the whole butt and almost nothing but the butt.

WARNING: If you find that squats or lunges are causing pain in your knees, STOP. Soreness is expected, but pain is an indication that you are doing them wrong or they're just wrong for you. When doing lunges, try not lowering so far and for Squats, move your feet further apart (toes out) and this should relieve the problem. But if it doesn't, stick with the Back Leg Exercises instead.

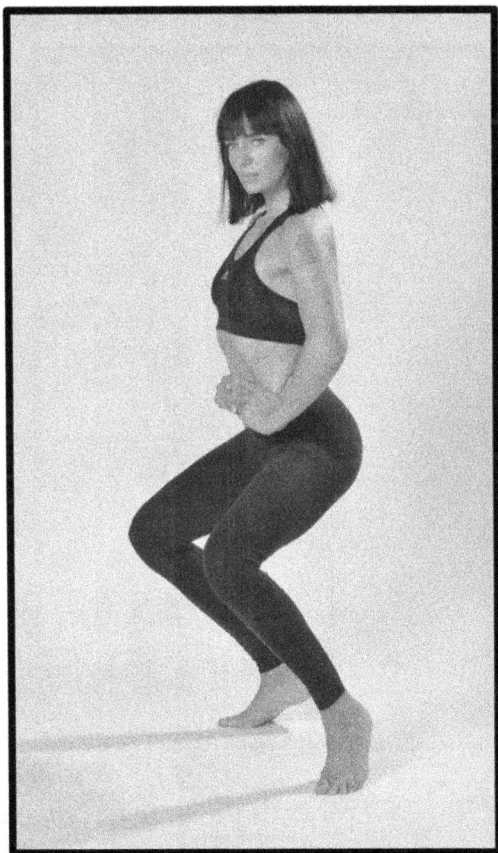

a) <u>Standard Squats</u>

(main muscles: butt, quads and hamstrings)

To work the most muscles, stand with your knees out past your shoulders. Place your hands on your hips (or raised out in front) as you bend your knees and lower your torso to almost a sitting position.

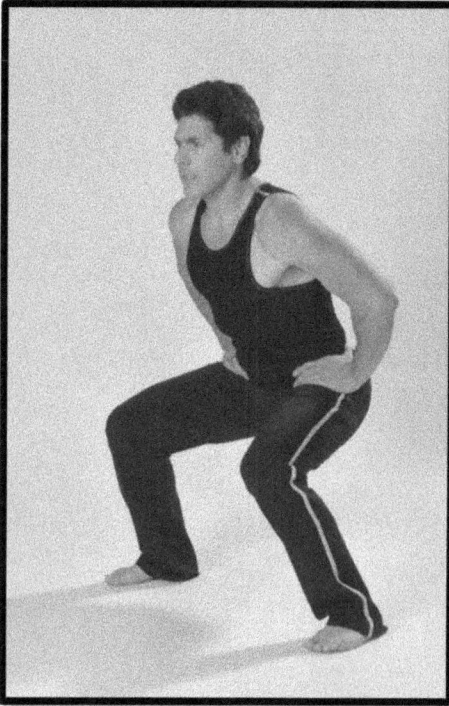

If you feel it too much on your knees and not enough in your butt, try widening your stance, like a Sumo wrestler. This will take some of the weight off your quads and shift it to your inner thighs.

Do this move for about two to three sets of ten reps, with a break between sets.

NOTE: *Lower until you feel it's the right level for you, concentrating on feeling it in your butt. You may not feel the full effects of this exercise right away, but you probably will tomorrow.*

b) <u>Medicine-Ball Wall Squats</u>

(main muscles: butt and quads)

Place a medicine ball between your back and a wall, just above your butt. Now, roll the ball up your back as you lower your torso down to a sitting position. The further apart your feet, the less your quads are worked with less stress on your knees and the more you'll use the muscles in your butt and also your thighs.

Try doing at least ten reps, rest and repeat for a total of three sets.

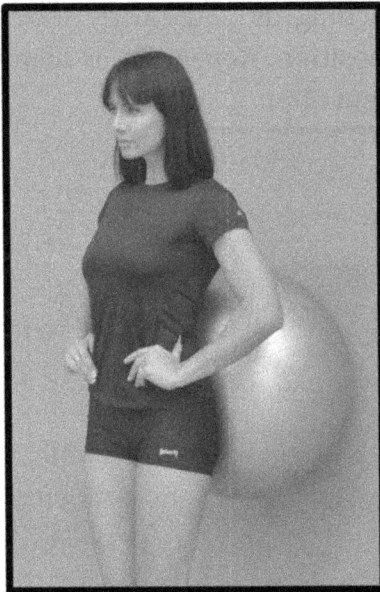

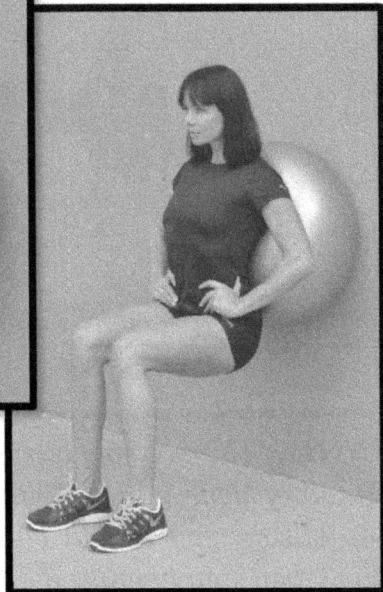

NOTE: While not as effective as a Standard Squat, it puts less strain on the knees.

c) <u>Chair Squats</u>*

(main muscles: butt, hamstrings, triceps and quads)

Using a chair (or any surface **THAT WON'T PUSH AWAY FROM YOU),** hover in front – halfway between the edge and the floor; supporting yourself from behind, with legs bent at about 90 degrees – as shown. Clench your butt and hamstrings as tight as possible, as you push up to the edge of the chair, *trying not to use your thighs and triceps.* Hold for a beat. Continue clenching as you slowly lower your body to the starting position. Repeat for as many reps as you can. And do them often.

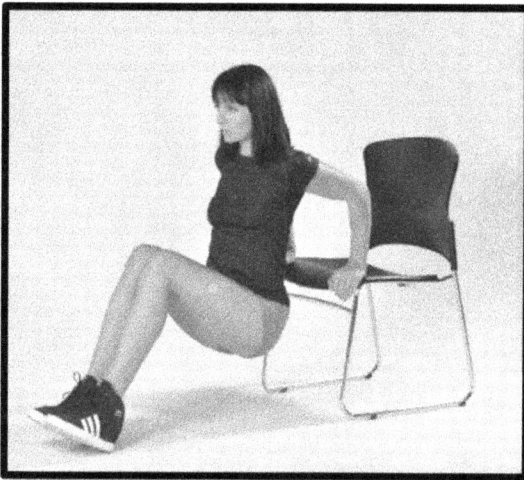

LEVEL I: #1 THE BUTT – e) Chair Butt Clench (Version #2) offers an alternate, non-moving version.

NOTE: *This is easily a triceps exercise that requires isolating your glutes. With a little effort and extra visualizing you should be able to do it. But if you can't then simply make it a triceps exercise. Just do it.*

d) <u>Standard Lunges</u>

(main muscles: glutes, quads and hamstrings)

With one leg slightly forward and bent at the knee, stretch your other leg back and lower your body half way to the floor, with your back knee as far down as you can go and still be able to get back up. Concentrate on tightening your butt cheek on the forward leg as you lower and raise. Now switch legs.

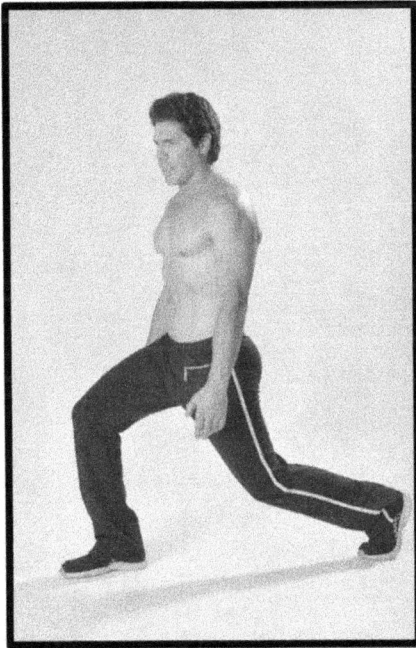

Work both legs evenly for at least three sets of ten reps each, always challenging yourself to do more.

Adjusting the distance between your feet changes how your quads and hamstrings are effected. It won't be painful but it may not be comfortable and that's the idea. Your butt has no doubt been far too comfortable for way too long.

NOTE: *Hands at your sides is best, but if needed, place them on the front knee for balance and support.*

e) <u>Kneeling Leg Lifts</u>

(main muscles: butt and hamstrings)

Kneel in front of an arm chair. Hold the chair with both hands and lift one leg up and back and hold, squeezing your butt. Leaning forward as you lift will increase your range of motion. Release, then lower for about ten reps. Repeat with the other leg. If you can do a few sets of these, do it.

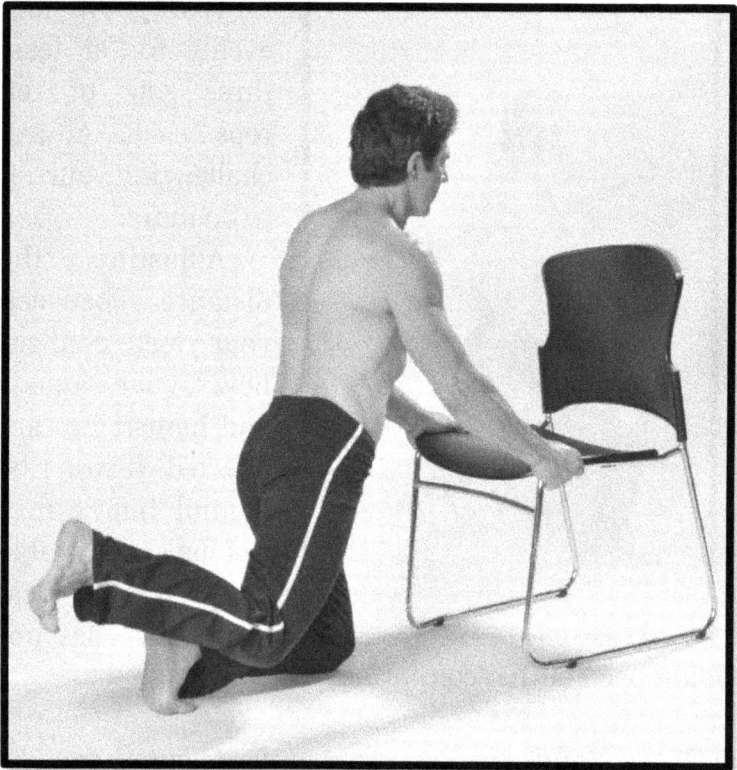

f) <u>Backward Leg Lifts</u>

(main muscles: butt, hamstring and lower back)

Version #1: While on your hands and knees, lift one leg up and back, bent at the knee at about a 90 degree angle. Really squeeze the butt muscle being lifted for a three-count and return for ten reps.

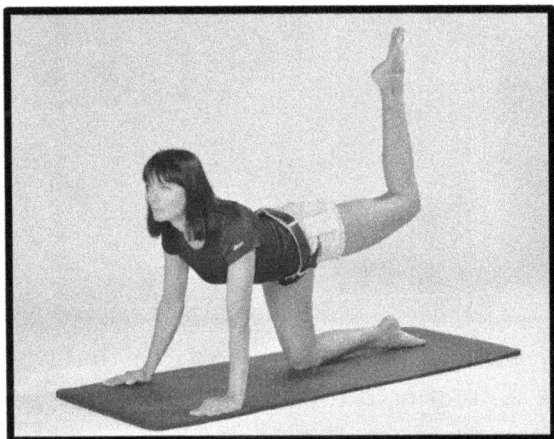

Repeat with your other leg. Three sets would be good.

Version #2: You can place even more emphasis on the butt by straightening your legs and while on your toes, lift one leg way up and back. If you still

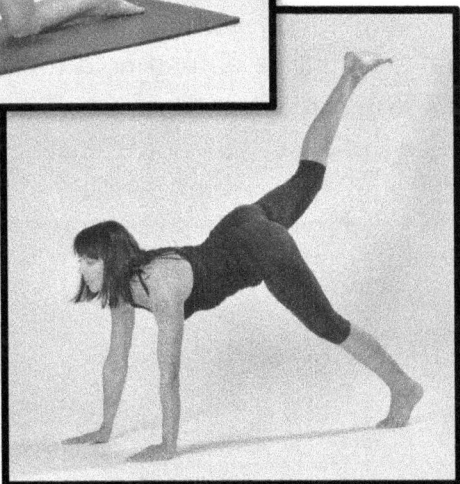

want more of a stretch, rest on your forearms as you lift each leg up. For this, you might want a mat.

g) <u>Medicine-Ball Backward Leg Lifts</u>

(main muscles: butt, lower back and hamstrings)

Facing forward, with your hands straight down on the floor, lay your mid-section on the medicine ball, with your legs straight back.

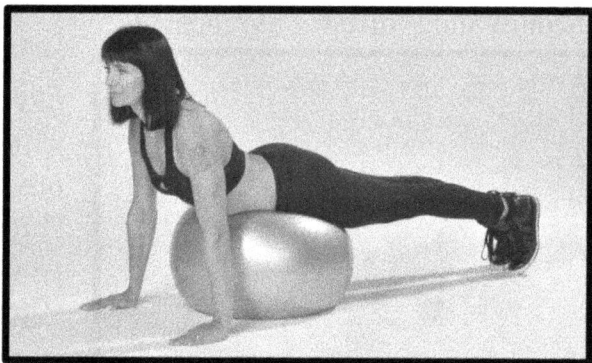

Roll forward slightly at the same time that you raise your legs up and hold for a couple seconds. Try to really squeeze your butt. Roll back and lower your legs slowly to the floor. Repeat for a total of ten reps, rest and do two more sets.

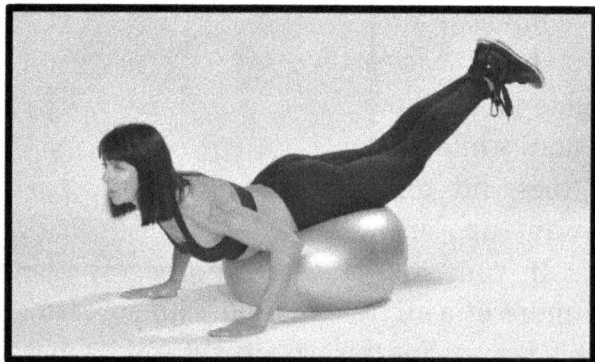

h) Medicine-Ball Plank

(main muscles: butt, hamstrings, abs and lower back)

While balancing on a medicine-ball and resting on your forearms, raise your legs until your body is angled as straight as possible – your head lower than your feet – using your butt and also your hamstrings. Hold this position for a ten count or as long as you're able, then release.

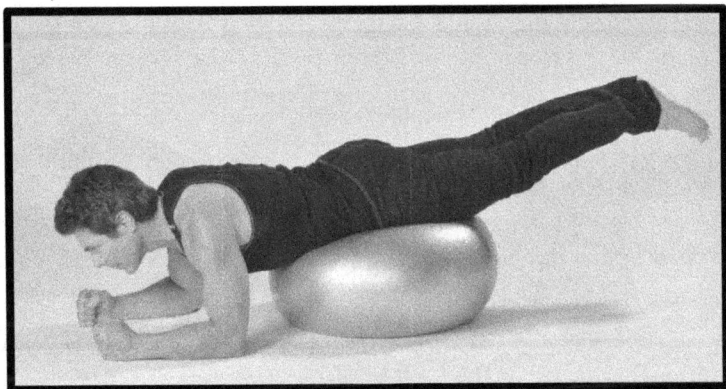

If you can do five to ten reps, do them. One set is pretty good, but do two more if you're up to the challenge.

NOTE: *Unlike The Plank that mainly works your stomach, the Medicine-Ball Plank targets your butt and back because your legs are held up off the floor. (see #2 STOMACH and THIGH EXERCISES - c) The Plank, in the next exercise group)*

i) <u>Superman</u>

(main muscles: butt, hamstrings and lower back)

While lying on your stomach, with your arms and legs outstretched, raise your extremities up as far as you can, trying to reach the sky backwards. Hold for at least three seconds as you tense your muscles. Lower and repeat. If you're up to it, do three sets, now or when time or opportunity allows.

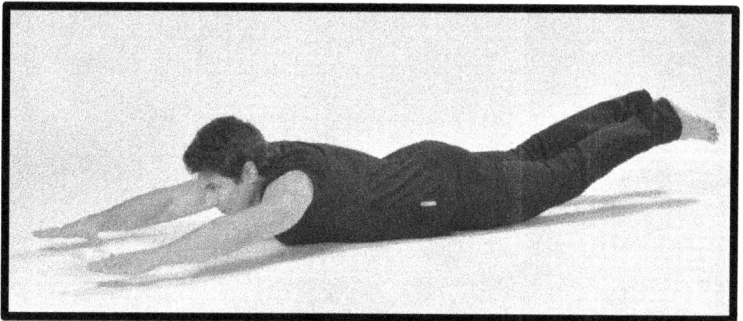

As you can see, Billy's position looks pretty much like Superman, without the cape.

Hint: One more time, we would like to recommend using a mat or some kind of padding to protect your joints, muscles and other "Superman" parts.

j) Stairway Butt Lifts

(main muscles: butt, hamstrings and quads)

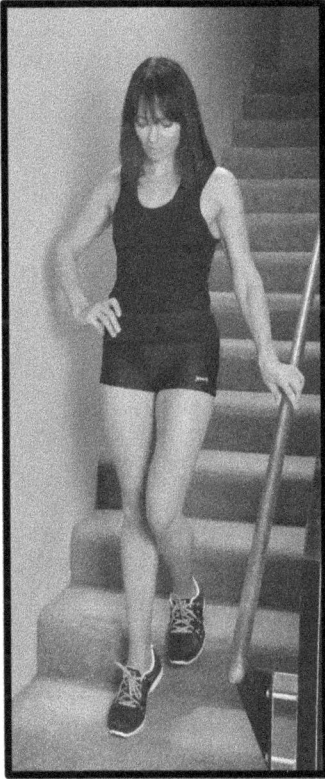

Moving forward – as you walk down a stairway or an incline, fully engage the butt cheek of your <u>straightened front leg</u>, while you lower onto each step. You may also find yourself clenching the upper back of that same leg – your hamstring. However, leaning back slightly as you plant your foot will isolate the butt even more. Step and clench. When walking up a stairway or an incline, this time at every step, pause for a moment and clench as hard as you can, on your <u>straightened back leg</u>.

Moving backward (<u>going up only</u>) – as you walk up backwards clench your glutes the same as walking up above, as you land with your <u>straightened back leg</u>.

WARNING: This exercise is not recommended for anyone who has difficulty walking or keeping their balance. If traversing a stairway, always hold onto a railing to prevent losing your balance and falling.

k) <u>Stairway Calf Lift</u>

(main muscles: calves)

Starting on the bottom step of a stairway, while holding on to a railing, step up, concentrating your effort on the calf of the leg doing the lifting.

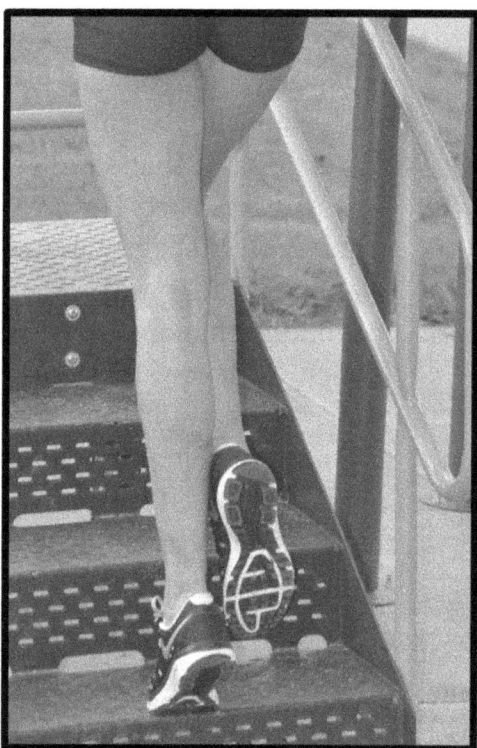

This works like a Rising Calf Clench, but with movement all through the clench. Again, ten reps are good, resting between sets. However, in this position you can get a really good stretch of the calf muscle, so you can safely use either one <u>or both calves</u> at a time, with little risk of cramping*.

*CAUTION: Still, be careful when tensing the calves <u>without resistance</u> just in case they cramp up, especially if you're not used to exercising.

#2 STOMACH and THIGH EXERCISES

These moves will mainly work your stomach. Don't worry about doing too much, just too little. And when you've done enough, you'll feel it. Then do some more.

We recommend that for all exercises you do while lying on your back, you use a mat or rug to cushion your spine. But avoid doing them on a bed, except for leg lifts, because it can negatively affect your results.

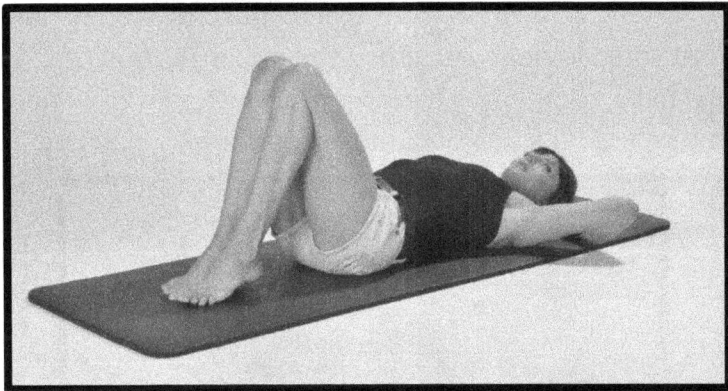

*WARNING: Placing your hands behind your head is fine but **do not** pull up with them as you crunch. This puts dangerous strain on your neck and spine.*

NOTE: *If you have an ab roller or similar device, feel free to use it for any of the applicable crunches or other applicable exercises in this section.*

HINT: If needed, hook your feet under an immovable object or have someone hold them in place.

a) <u>Standard Crunch</u>

(main muscles: upper abs)

Lie on your back, with your knees up and head elevated slightly – your fingers touching behind your ears (BUT DON'T PULL FROM BEHIND YOUR HEAD). The more bent and higher your knees, the more your upper abs will be worked.

Trying to use your stomach muscles alone, raise your torso enough to crunch the upper portion of your abs hard, then lower back down to just above the floor and repeat. It's not a big move but it's very effective.

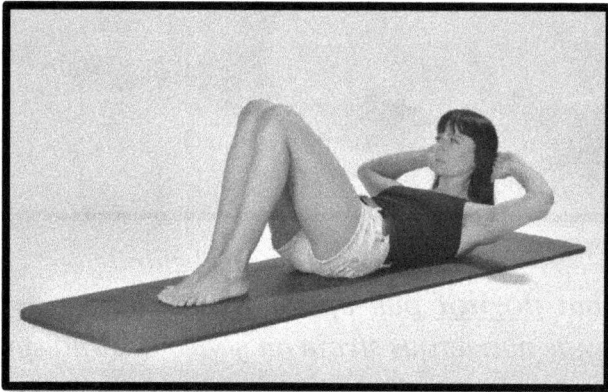

Unlike old-fashioned Sit Ups, where we tried to bend ourselves in half, a crunch moves a short distance and accentuates the stomach muscles more with little or no stress. See if you can do this about thirty to fifty times, rest and do two more sets, now or throughout your day. But whenever you do them, only do what you can. And as always, if you feel dizzy, stop.

b) <u>Standard Crunch (with a twist)</u>

(main muscles: obliques and upper abs)

This exercise is basically performed the same as the Standard Crunch, but this time twist your torso to one side at a time as you rise, turning your elbows toward your opposite knees. You'll probably find that your torso will rise higher than a Standard Crunch to have the best effect. Again, this is a fairly slight move, but effective. Do at least twenty crunches on each side without a break between them. Rest between sets (done consecutively or throughout your day).

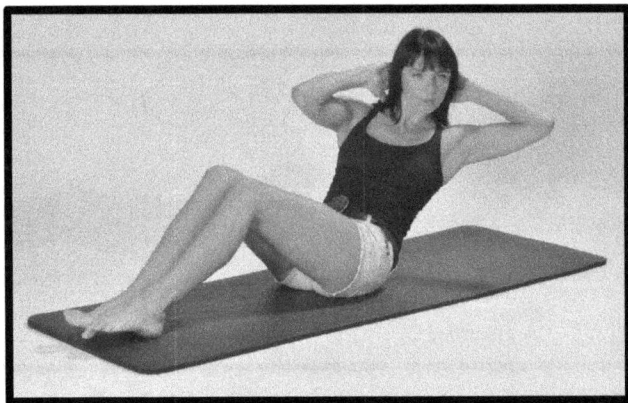

Alternate Version (not shown): With one knee up, cross the other leg (out to one side; its ankle over the raised knee) and crunch up, opposite elbow to side knee. You may find it works your obliques even better.

NOTE: *Choose the version that feels best to you and also feels the most effective in working your obliques.*

c) <u>The Plank</u>

(main muscles: shoulders, abs and lower back)

Starting face-down on the floor, hold up your torso with your forearms and raise your lower body up on your forward-bent toes, into a stationary, straight, prone position. Hold and firmly tighten your stomach, lower back and shoulders for a thirty-count, which may seem like forever, at the time. Lower, take a break and repeat. If you can do this for three reps, you're doing great. And if you can do another set – now or throughout your day – you are doing incredible.

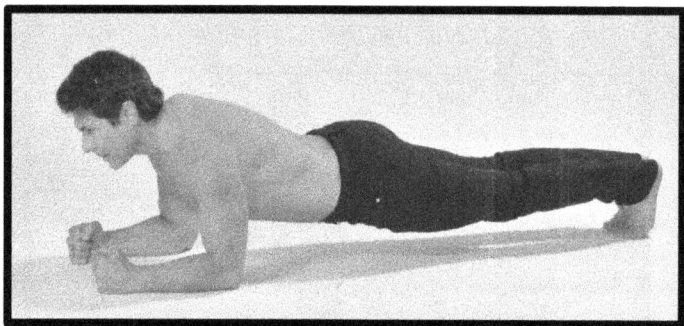

This exercise is a lot harder than it looks. In order to do it properly almost your whole body must be rigid. Even though the abs, lower back and shoulders are the main muscles used, you'll find it works just about every muscle you have to some extent.

NOTE: *It's probably best to do this on a mat, regardless of what Billy does or doesn't do.*

d) The Twisting Plank

(main muscles: obliques, back, shoulders and quads)

Starting from The Plank position, turn your body to one side with your arm and torso as straight up as possible and hold for five to fifteen seconds. One set of three reps (with breaks) will be hard, but worth trying. Just make sure you work both sides equally.

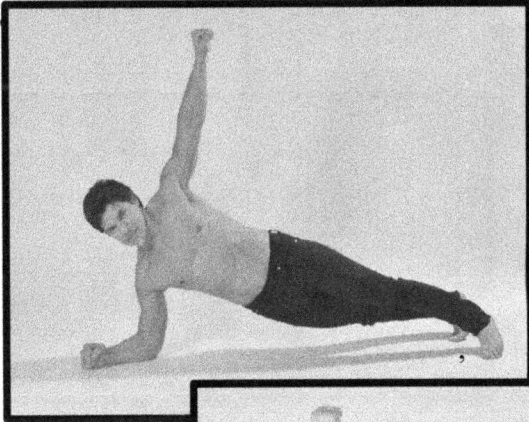

Hint: A mat just might be a good idea.

As you can see from the back, a lot of muscles are used in this one.

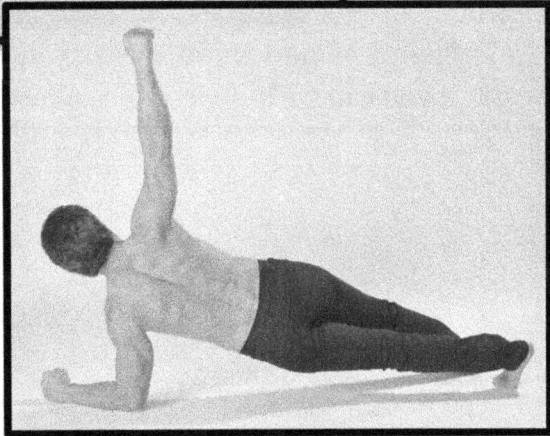

NOTE: *This isn't a substitute for The Plank. Try alternating with it for a more complete workout.*

e) <u>Forward Leg Lifts (lying down)</u>

(main muscles: abs and quads)

   While lying on your back, with your legs straight
and your hands palms-down, under your butt – or

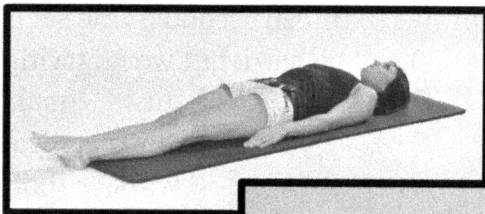

close to it –
raise your legs
up to about a 45
degree angle.

   Hold a few
seconds, lower
to about a foot
off the floor,
hold again and
repeat.

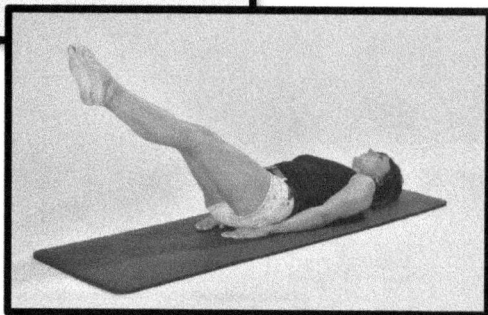

   Do ten reps and three sets if you can, but don't
worry if you can't. This exercise is effective, not easy.

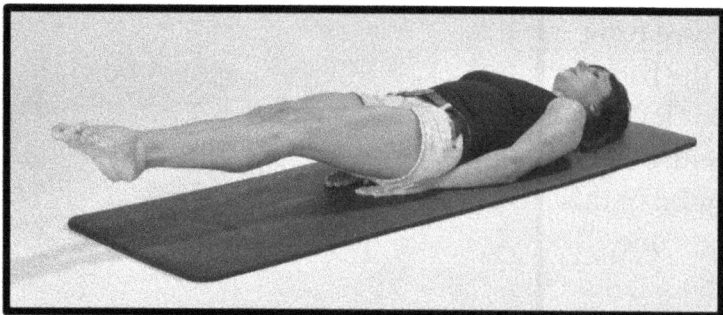

NOTE: *If holding between positions is too difficult
then try the above as continuous movements.*

f) Forward Leg Lifts (sitting)

(main muscles: lower abs and quads)

Version #1: Do these on any seat you can grip tightly. Start with your legs straight out and down, then bring your knees up toward your chest and return.

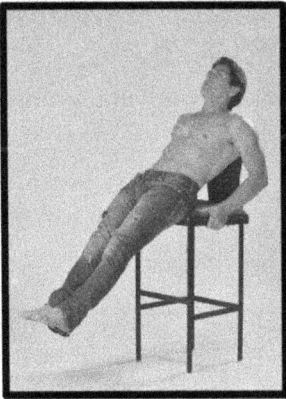

Try for at least twenty reps for three sets, but you can probably do more.

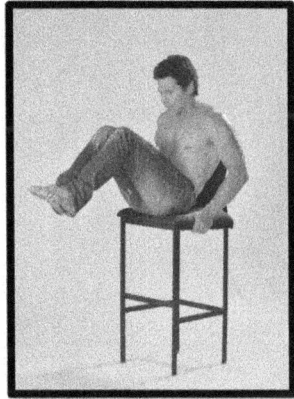

Version #2: Raise your legs parallel to the floor or higher if possible, hold, then return. This works your quads too, so isolate your abs the best you can.

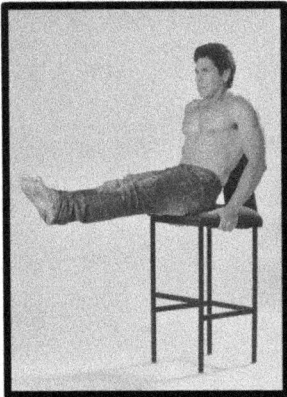

These are a little harder, so three sets of ten reps is good.

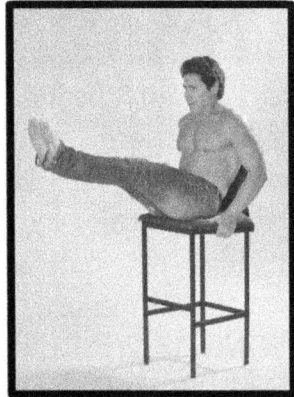

g) Stairway Thigh Lifts

(main muscles: quads and glutes)

This exercise is best done when going up a stairway rather than going down. That way, it's easier to isolate the thigh from the hamstrings and it's safer.

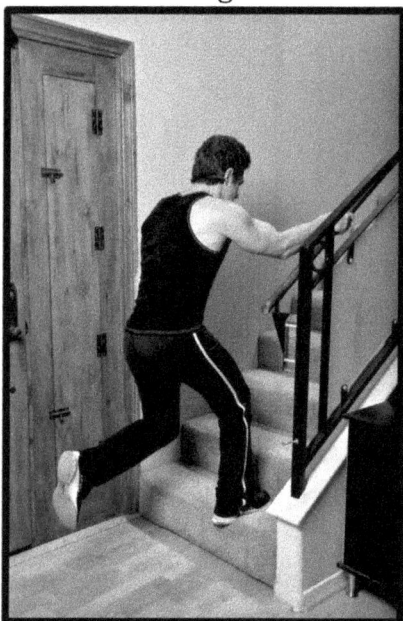

WHILE HOLDING THE RAILING, lean back – one leg angled behind you – and rise up to the next step as you clench hard with your forward thigh.

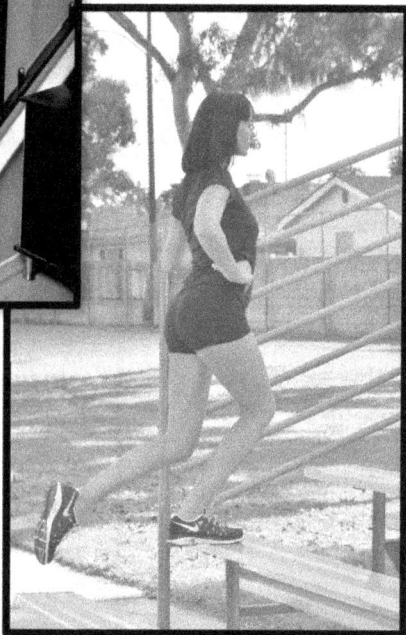

You won't be able to isolate your thighs completely, but keep trying, all the way up. Inside or out, it's worth the effort, AS LONG AS THERE IS A HAND RAILING.

#3 PUSH-UPS

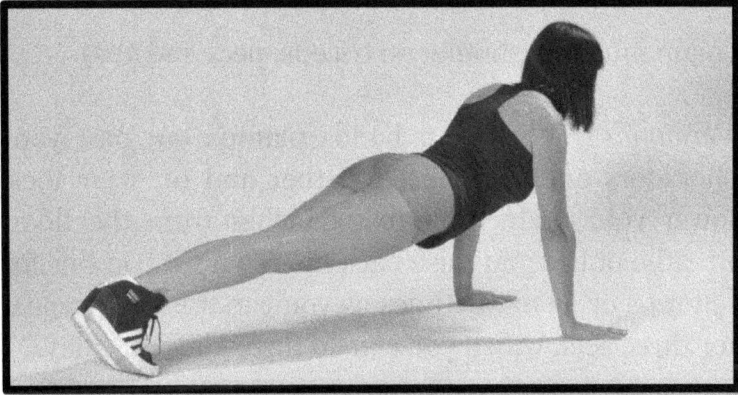

There are no better exercises than push-ups. Depending on your hand and feet positions they will work quite a few different muscles. For instance:

1. The wider your hands are placed, the more your chest is worked. The narrower your hands are placed the more your triceps are worked.

2. The placement of your feet directly affects your abs – the wider they're placed, the more the abs are worked as you stabilize your core.

Generally, when doing almost any Push-Up, be sure to keep your core as tight and body as rigid as you can, making sure your butt is not raised high. The proper form makes all the difference.

NOTE: *More intense push-ups can be found in* *LEVEL III: Muscle Resistance.*

a) <u>Standard Push-Ups</u>

(main muscles: shoulders; triceps, pecs and abs)

Version #1: With your hands planted out past your shoulders and your feet together and on your toes, lower your body three-to-six inches from the floor. Breathe out as you raise back up. That's it. Do this for ten reps or as many times as you can, rest and repeat for three sets, which you can do throughout the day.

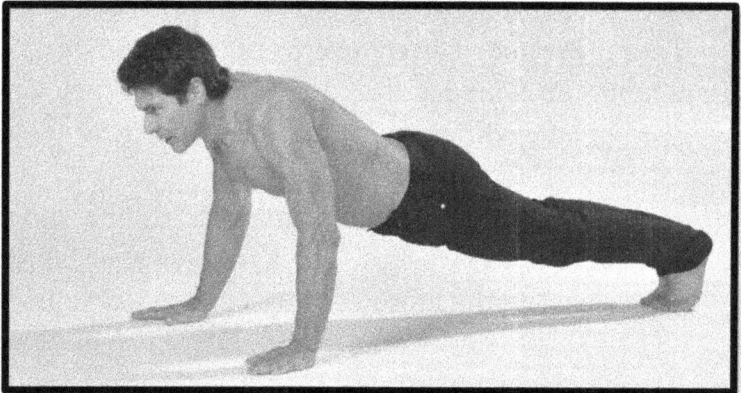

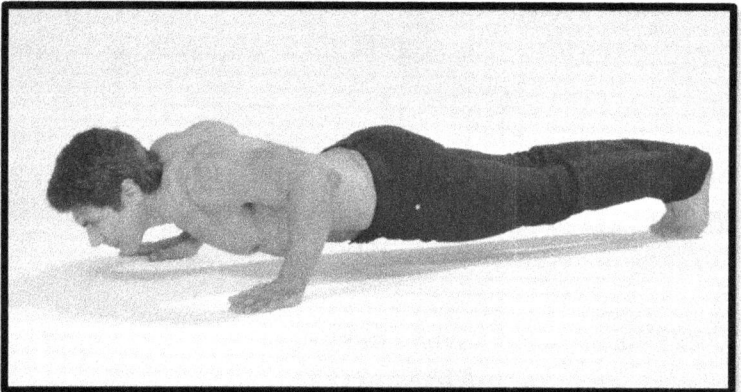

Version #2: The only real difference between this and Version #1 is that Inara's feet are further apart, which stabilizes her core as she works her abs.

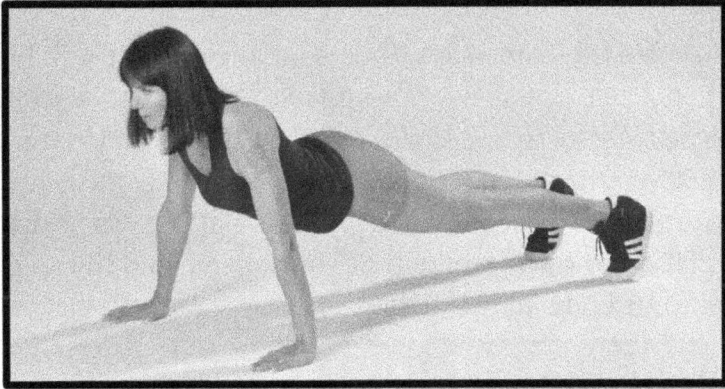

But basically, it's just a good excuse for shots of Inara.

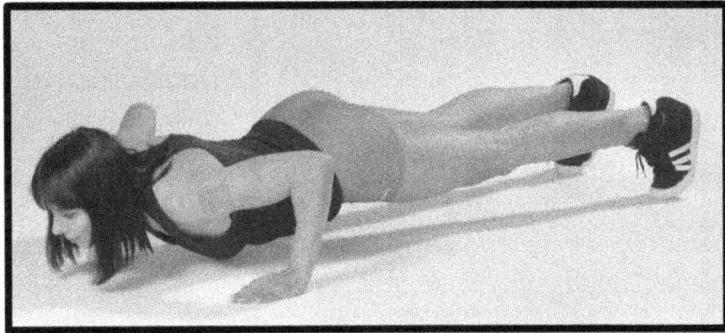

And one more, from a different angle, can't hurt.

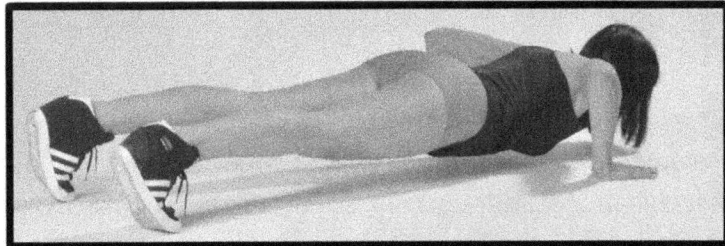

b) <u>Angled Push-Ups</u>

(main muscles: pecs, shoulders and triceps)

Like the name says, this is an angled push-up, but it doesn't involve your full body weight and is especially good for those people who haven't done a push-up in a long time. And as with all push-ups, your chest, triceps and shoulders will be worked in relation to the placement of your hands and the angle of your body to the floor.

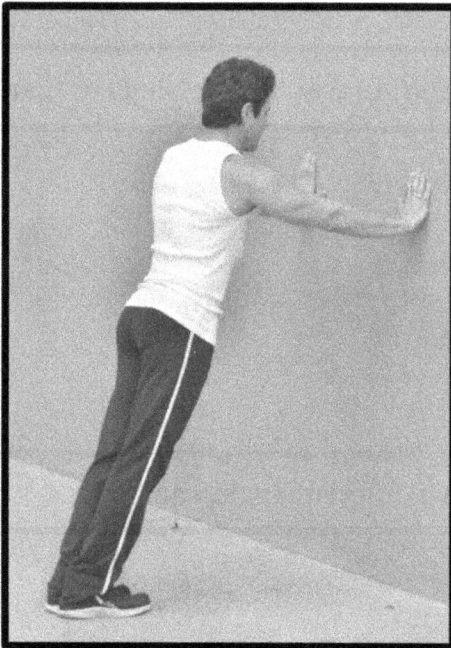

NOTE: *This exercise can be done at a desk, a counter, a wall or any immovable object. Just remember, <u>the closer your chest is to the floor, the harder the push-up.</u>*

Keeping your hands closer together works your triceps more and moving them farther apart works your shoulders more, but they all will work your chest.

With your hands on the resisting object, place your feet together or apart (your choice) and as far away from the resisting object as you feel comfortable. Keeping your back straight, lean your body all the way forward and push all the way back, CLENCHING YOUR CHEST THROUGH THE WHOLE MOVE.

BONUS: If you truly want this exercise to be its most beneficial, try doing some reps while also, <u>or mainly</u>, clenching your hamstrings, thighs, glutes, lats, triceps or abs. And not just clench, but really clench. You may find this kind of push-up actually allows you to engage them more than the muscles that this exercise was primarily designed to engage in the first place. You might as well get the most out of it that you can. So, clench them all!

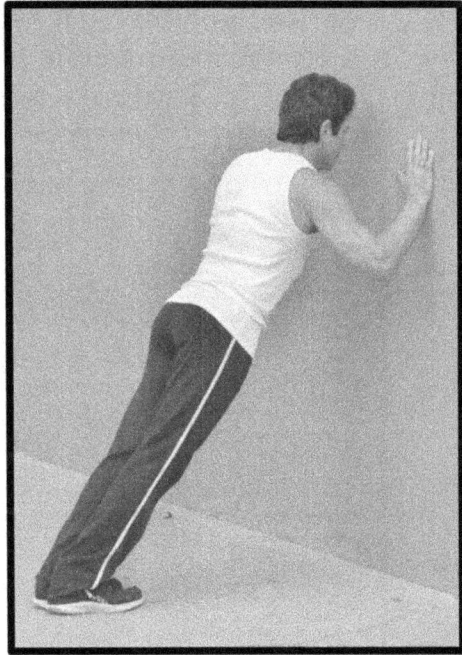

WARNING: Be extra careful to always plant your feet securely so your legs will not slip out from under you.

c) <u>Modified Push-Ups</u>

(main muscles: shoulders, triceps and pecs)

Position your hands the same as for Standard Push-Ups (wide or narrow), but this time, bend from your knees as you lower your torso to the floor with your feet crossed and raised in the air. If you can, do more than ten reps for three sets now, or over the day.

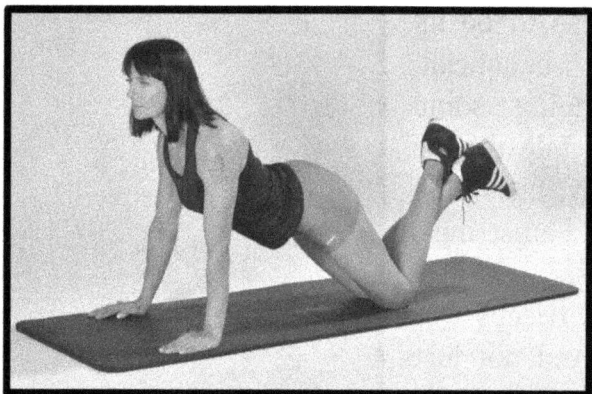

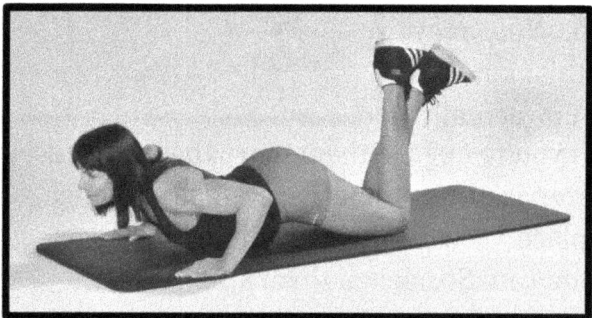

NOTE: *This exercise works your muscles less than other Push-Ups, but it does work. So, if you're having trouble doing the others, this is the one to try.*

#4 CURLS, LIFTS and PUSHES

Whenever you work your upper arms or shoulders, or even your chest, you'll find that one or the other is also worked to some extent. They are hard muscles to completely isolate, but you don't really have to. Just be aware of it and with a little practice you can zero in on the muscle group you're trying to highlight.

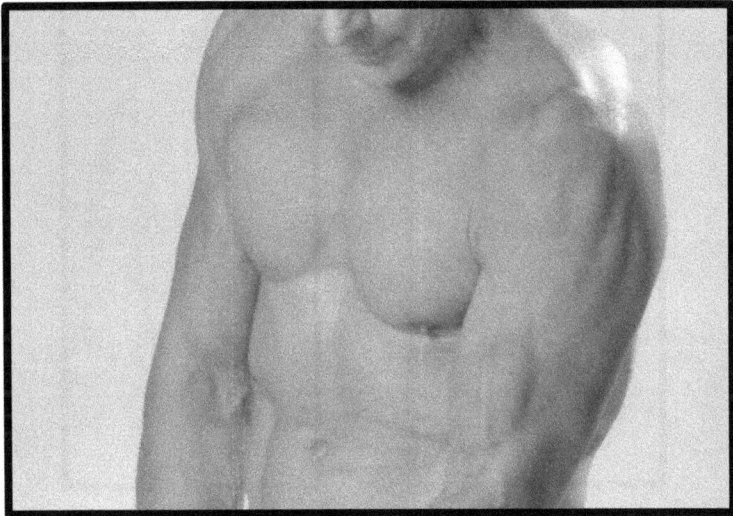

a) <u>Band Curls</u>

(main muscles: biceps and shoulders)

Either standing or sitting, start with your forearm down by your side or at a 90 degree angle as shown (try doing both ways to vary your workout), curl the gripped band to your chest, lower and repeat.

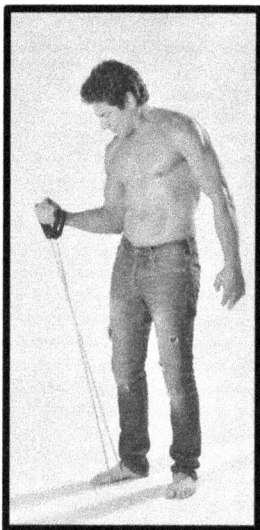

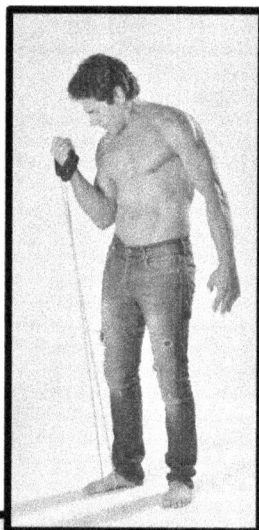

WARNING: For your safety, be sure the band is secured under your feet or an immovable object. And as always, if you feel <u>any</u> twinges, STOP.

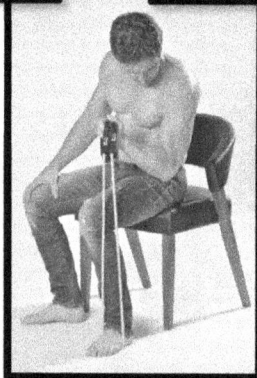

NOTE: Try ten reps for three sets on each arm. If that's too easy, use a stronger band or do more.

b) <u>Freestyle Curls</u>

(main muscles: biceps and chest)

Using one arm for pulling and the other for resisting, extend one arm down at your side; fist facing up. Place your other hand over the fist of your extended arm. Clench the target bicep and with a steady motion, curl it up toward your shoulders, resisting with your other arm the whole way. And you'll definitely feel the burn.

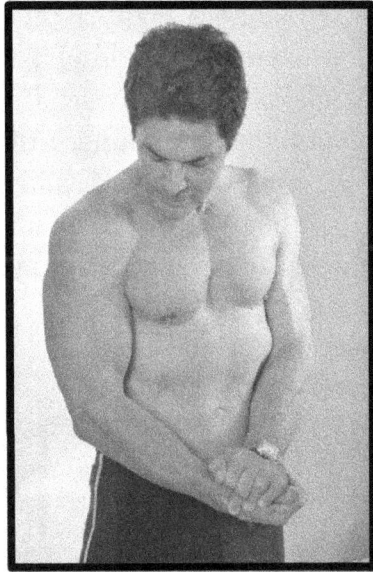

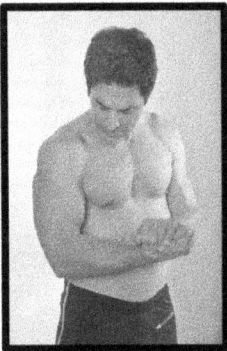

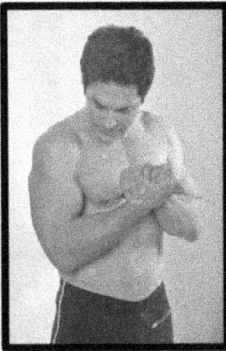

At the top of the curl, hold the clench for a three count. Try to do this for ten reps and three sets <u>on each arm</u> equally.

NOTE: *The triceps and lats of the resisting arm will also be worked but not as much as the biceps.*

c) <u>Freestyle Lifts</u>

(main muscles: biceps, shoulders, lats, chest and abs)

In lieu of weights, you can use almost anything for this exercise; anything you can grip in one or both hands and lift – or curl. Chairs work well. So do sacks of potatoes, containers of water, laundry detergent, your infant child (lift safely), even large cans of food.

Either work your shoulders more by holding the **object further away from your body as you lift** or work your biceps more by keeping the object* close as you curl.

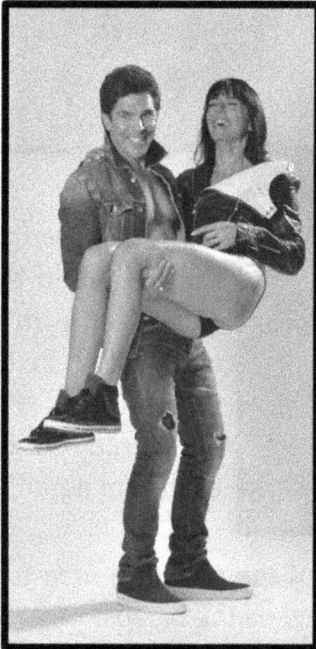

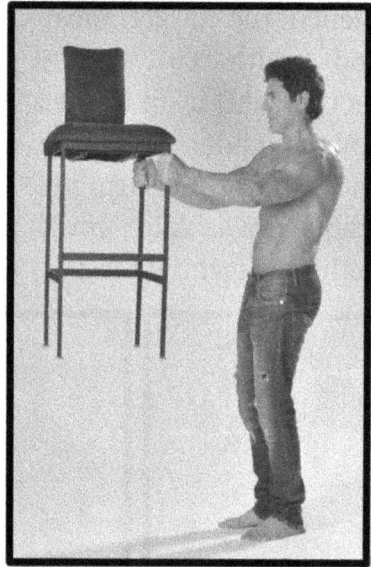

Sometimes Billy's choice for a curling object is questionable, plus he's cheating with Inara's arm around his shoulders.

d) <u>Triceps Push</u>

(main muscles: triceps, lats and pecs)

While standing inside of a waist-high, counter corner, place your hands on the edge of the counter at your sides. Raise yourself off of the floor, engaging your triceps. <u>Lower only as far as you feel comfortable</u> and return (or hold a clench at your lowest point). Do as many reps as you can without straining.

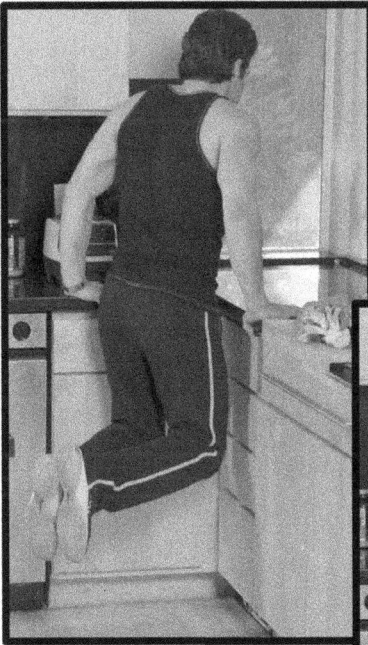

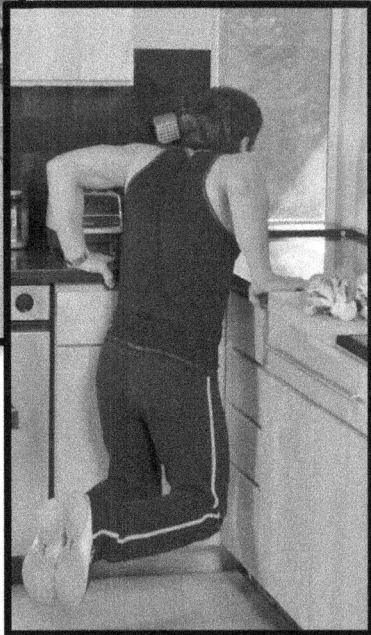

BONUS: By engaging your abs, you can get quite a good workout on them at the same time. And any time you can work your abs is the right time to do it.

e) <u>Forearm Push</u>

(main muscles: forearms)

This exercise works much the same way as the Freestyle Curl and is an extension of the Freestyle Forearm Clench. With one arm down at your waist, make a fist with that hand (fingers up). Place your other hand over your fist and move the wrist of that fist in an upward motion – trying to isolate your forearm – while resisting with your other hand. Then turn your fist around (fingers down) and repeat the upward motion, resisting again with your other hand. Work both wrists equally for about five reps and three sets, or until you feel it. This move can be done either standing or sitting, whichever you prefer.

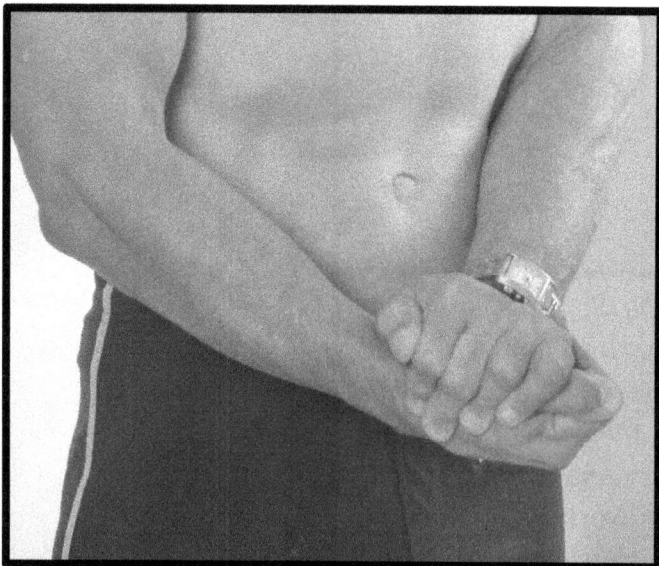

f) Chest "Rope Pull"*

(main muscles: chest, biceps and triceps)

This move may look like you are *pulling* on an imaginary rope but it is actually a *pushing* motion, that works each side of your chest semi-individually.

Clenching your chest, place one fist on top of the other at shoulder height and push down with the top fist while resisting with the bottom fist. As you move both fists down to your waist (or back up), the *pushing* side of your chest will always be dominant.

Now, switch the position of your fists at your waist. Return them to your shoulders by pushing up with your bottom fist and resisting with your top fist.

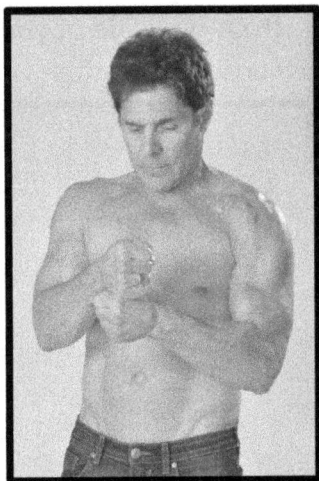

*pictures taken 2017

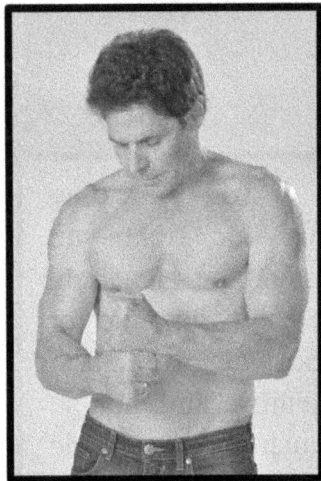

Be sure to work both sides of your chest evenly and try to do ten reps for three sets.

g) <u>Chest Push</u>

(main muscles: pecs, biceps and triceps)

Like the "Rope Pull", this exercise greatly isolates your pecs but still utilizes your triceps and biceps.

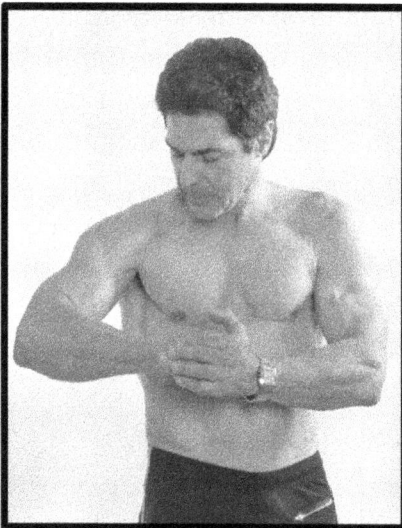

Bend one arm at the elbow and out to the side, with your forearm parallel to your shoulders. Place the palm of your other hand over your fisted hand and resist as you push your fist from one side of your chest to the other.

If you are doing this one right you should be clenching mainly the side of your chest doing the pushing and not so much the side resisting. Do the move for ten reps on each side, for three sets each.

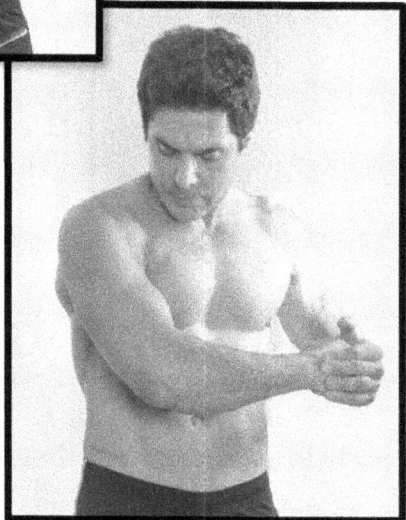

h) <u>Shoulders Lift</u>*

(main muscles: shoulders)

With your arms at 90 degree angles (using bands held just above the shoulders), slowly push up as high as you can. Hold for a beat and then slowly return to the start position. Try for ten reps and three sets.

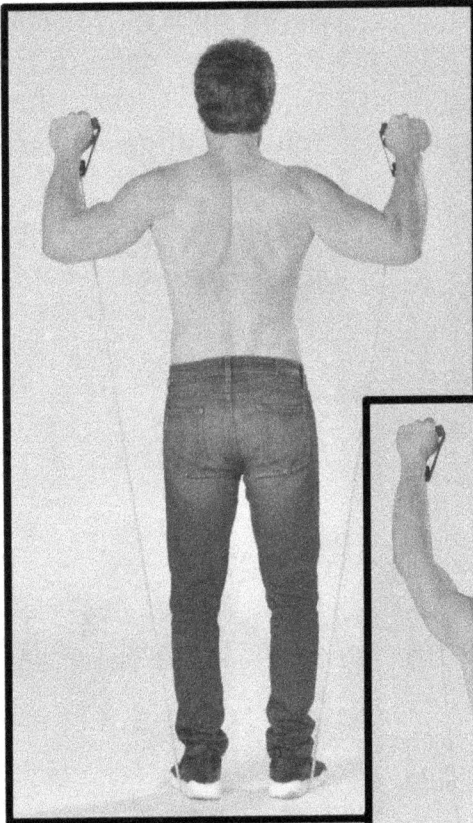

NOTE: *Use a band strong enough to give good resistance, but doesn't cause strain.*

*pictures taken 2017

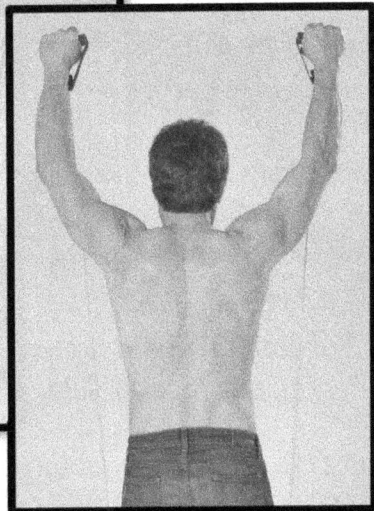

<u>Strong Reminder</u>: Make sure the band is secure.

i) <u>Moving Lats Lift</u>

(main muscles: lats, triceps and pecs)

While sitting in a chair with arm rests, grip the arms and slowly raise yourself up, trying your best to isolate your lats. At the top of the move, clench hard and hold. Release as you lower back down. Try for ten reps – or as many as you can until you are able to really feel it – whenever you find yourself sitting around.

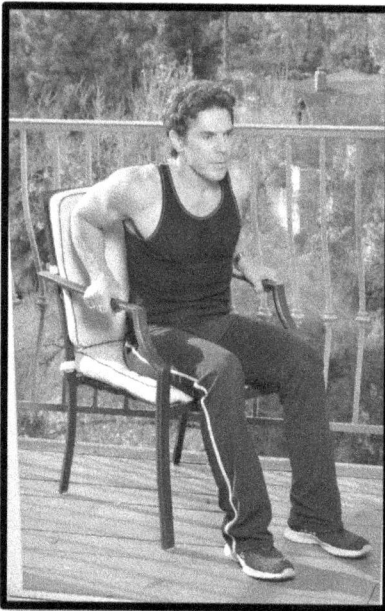

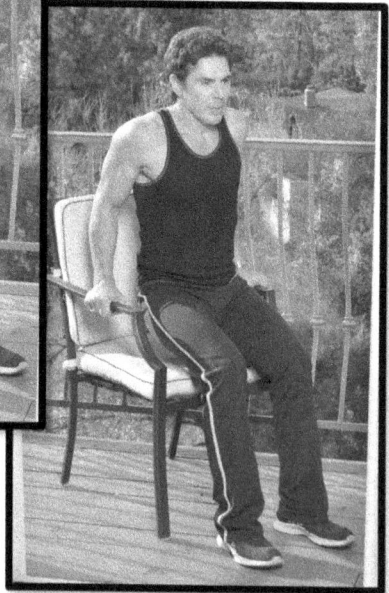

It's a good excuse for bobbing up and down over your office cubicle.

NOTE: *This is a moving version of the LEVEL I: #5 THE UPPER BACK – b) Lats Lift Clench*

j) Medicine-Ball Neck Lifts

(main muscles: neck)

While lying on a medicine-ball (butt to shoulders – your legs forward and bent at the knees), balance with your hands and feet as you raise and lower your neck.

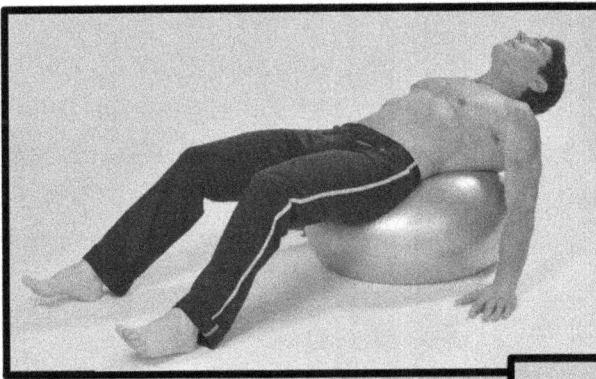

NOTE: the average head weighs about ten pounds.

Also, do the same move with your head turned to the right and left.

A great exercise, especially if you work at a desk.

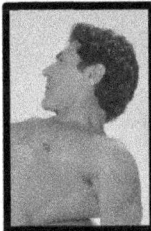

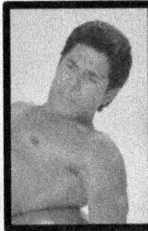

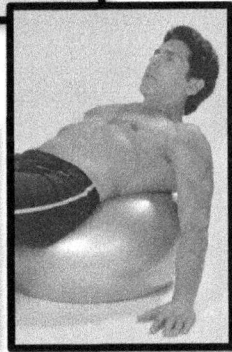

Do these moves for about ten reps each and three sets and you'll get results, one of which is probably a better night's sleep.

Alternate Method: This move can also be performed on a bed with your head hanging over the edge.

#5 AEROBICS

Aerobics get your blood flowing and your heart pumping. For LEVEL II we recommend taking a brisk walk, going for a light jog or cruising around on a bike.

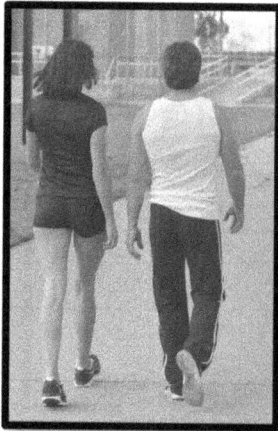

You don't have to go berserk, just get moving, take your time and work up to something more active when you're ready.

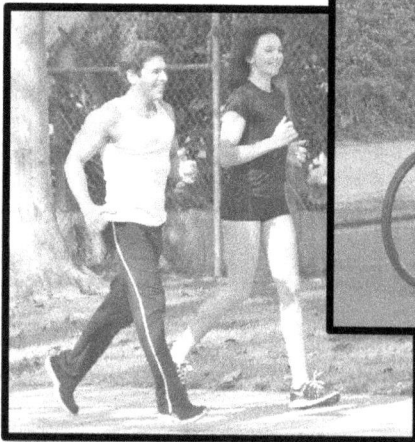

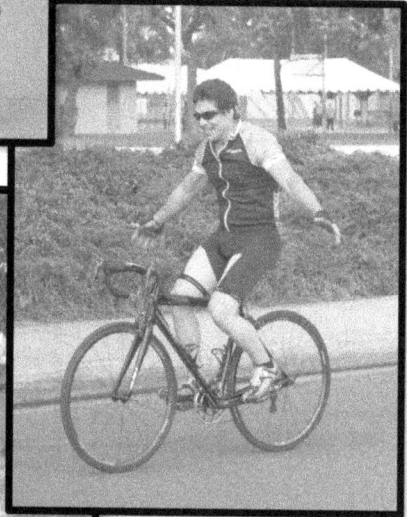

You can also perform one of the following simple exercises that involve mainly stationary movement.

a) <u>Basic Hopping</u>

(main muscles: whole body)

This is just what it sounds like – hopping. Simply hop on two feet or alternate between the two, as high as you safely can. If you start getting dizzy or winded, then stop. Otherwise keep hopping. After you've taken a break and caught your breath try hopping for three sets total, if you can.

Hint: As an added isometric workout, try to keep your abs and pecs clenched, as you hop.

NOTE: *Just a few inches off the floor is fine. Or go for more...*

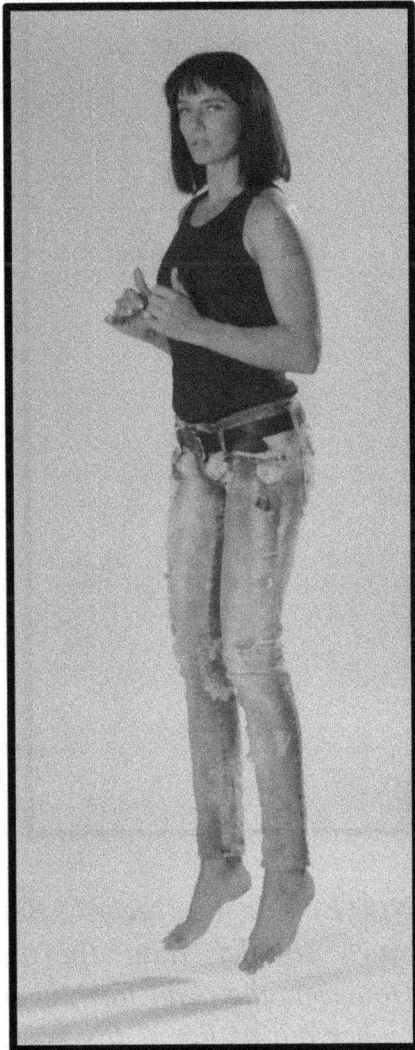

...like Inara...

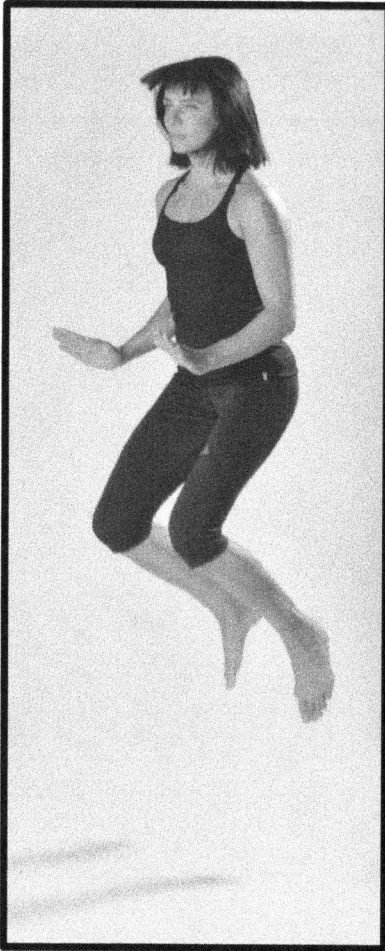

...or even, Billy. You decide.

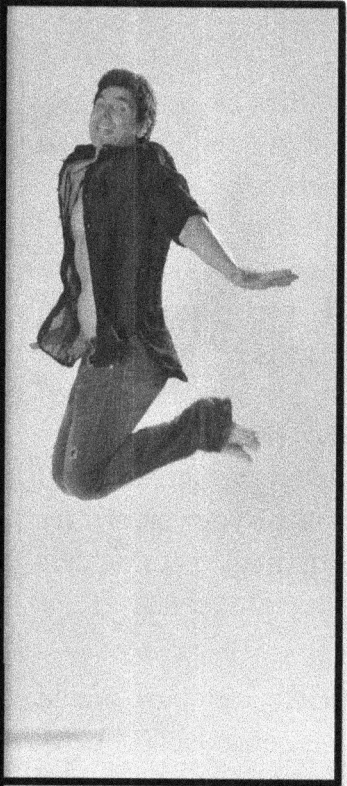

Hint: Just have fun. And don't overdo it.

NOTE: *For the record, Billy is not actually that much smaller than Inara. It's just an illusion. However, the right form is everything. Billy may be higher but as far as his execution goes... well... we'll let the picture speak for itself.*

b) <u>Imaginary Jump Rope</u>

(main muscles: whole body)

For an extra cardio workout beyond Basic Hopping try using an "imaginary jump rope". As you hop up and down, swing your arms out and around as you jump over your pretend rope.

Like Basic Hopping, do this as much as you can, take a break and then do some more. You'll know when you've had enough.

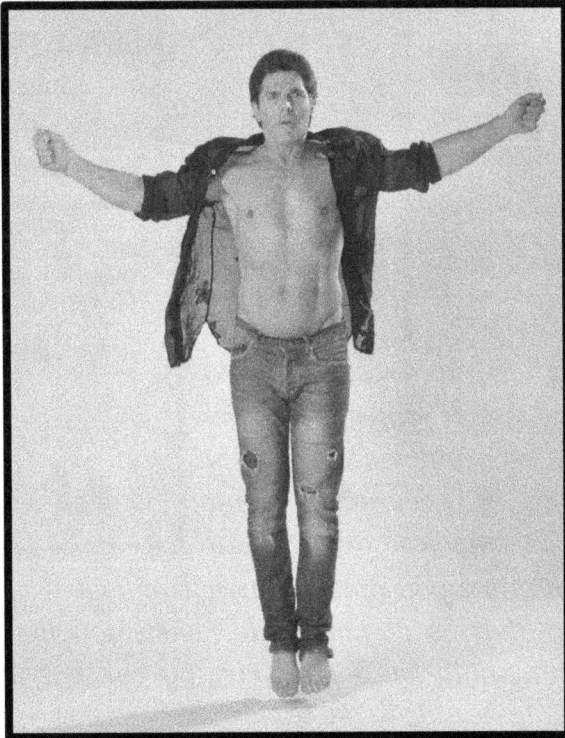

c) <u>Jumping Jacks</u>

(main muscles: whole body)

Start with your feet together and arms at your sides. Jump up and out wide with your feet, simultaneously swinging your arms out and up until they meet at the top. Without stopping, jump up and swing back to the starting position – hands at sides; feet together – and continue your workout in this manner for about fifteen seconds or longer. It'll really get your heart pumping.

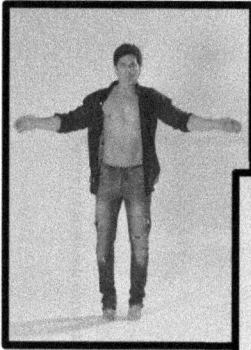

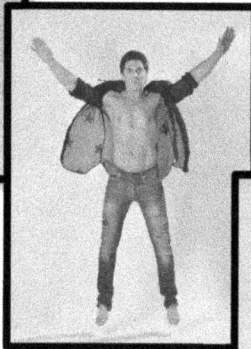

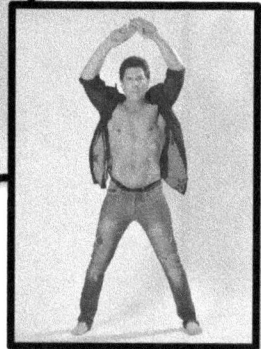

NOTE: This exercise works best if you can raise your arms and move your legs correctly. However, if you are having trouble raising your arms up at the same time you move your legs out then you can keep your arms at your side, when you jump. It's better than nothing. But keep trying, concentrate and you should be able to get it.

#6 STRETCHING

Like all things in life, when we push a little harder to do something, we increase our ability to do it. Muscles react the same. Stretching improves muscle elasticity and gives us an increased range of motion.

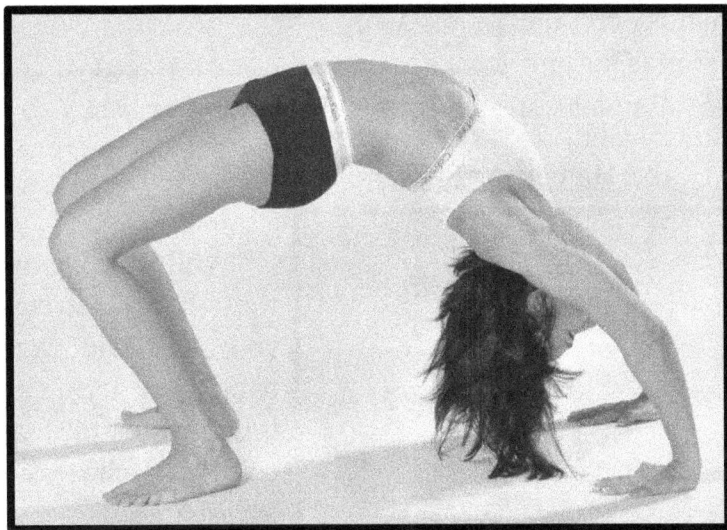

There are two types of stretching: Static Stretching (above) – holding a stretch for fifteen to thirty seconds or more; and Dynamic Stretching – slowly stretching through a range of motion. Either way, since stretching is actually an exercise, we suggest you do it at the end of your workout or throughout your day.

A WORD OF CAUTION: The "Exorcist" stretch above is extreme. Sometimes Inara is nutty, too. So, the rule is, "If it's painful, don't do it." Muscles can only stretch so far, so do so slowly and carefully.

a) Glutes/Lower Back Stretch

Resting on your knees, bend forward with your hands on the floor as far out as possible to stretch your glutes and lower back.

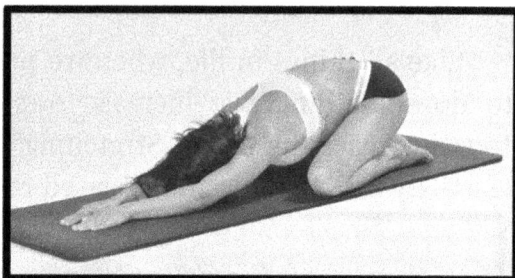

b) Hamstring Stretch

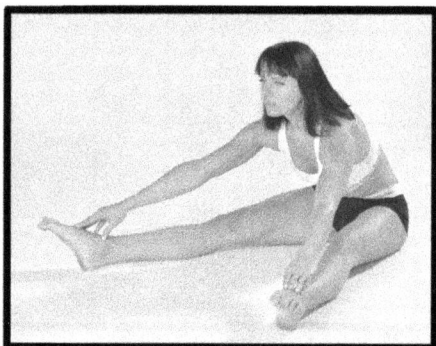

While sitting on the floor, stretch your legs wide and bend over trying to touch your toes as you stretch your hamstrings.

c) Quad Stretch - 1

Laying on your back, pull one leg toward your torso as far as you can and stretch your quad, with your bent knee as flat to the floor as possible.

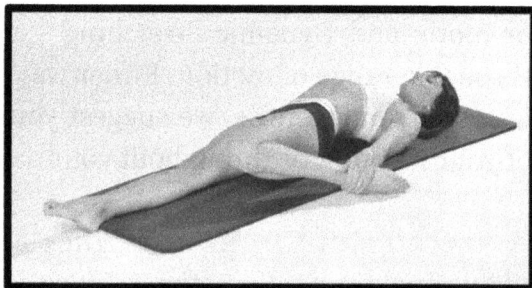

d) <u>Quad Stretch - 2</u>

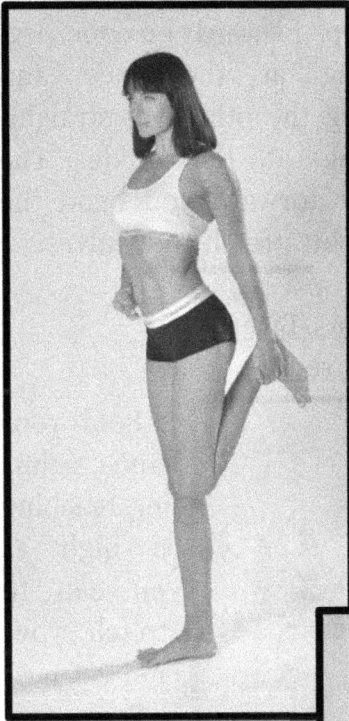

Balancing on one foot, pull your other foot back toward your butt to stretch your quad. And remember, the idea is to stretch.

e) <u>Inner Thigh Stretch</u>

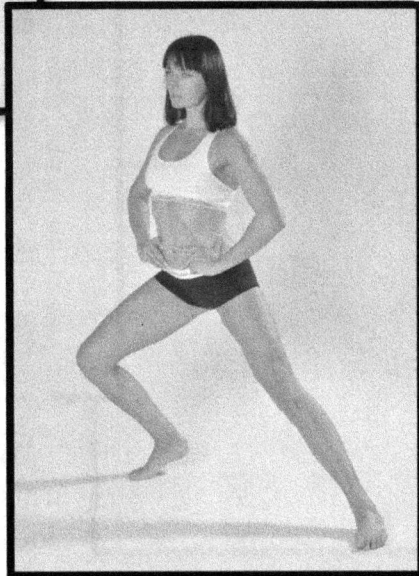

This is kind of a sideways lunge. With your feet and legs wide, bend toward one knee, keeping the other leg straight as you stretch its inner thigh.

f) Calf Stretch

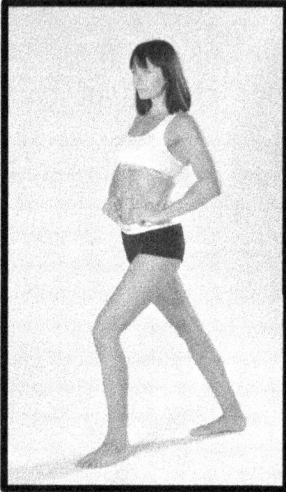

Step forward on one leg, bending at the knee and keeping the other leg straight, bending at the ankle. The further forward you bend the more you stretch your calves.

g) Lats/Biceps Stretch

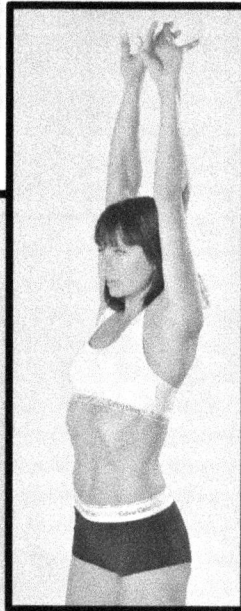

Fold your hands, palms up, reaching as high as you can to stretch your lats.

Squeezing your arms further to your head and back will also stretch your biceps.

h) Obliques Stretch

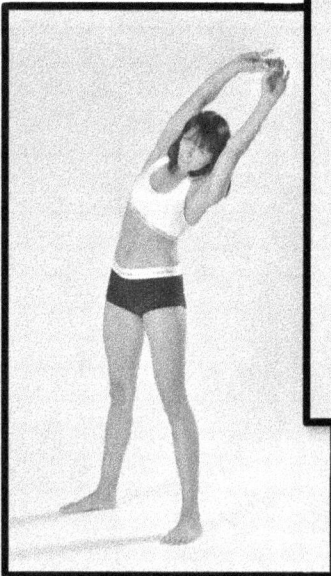

With feet apart and arms straight up, bend sideways at the waist – to each side – to stretch your obliques.

i) <u>Shoulder Stretch</u>

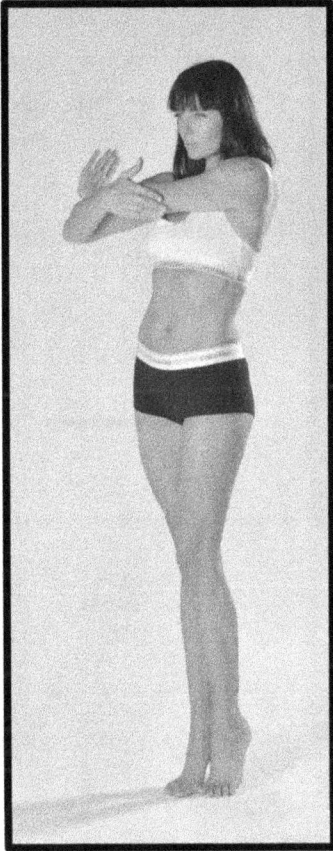

j) <u>Chest Stretch</u>

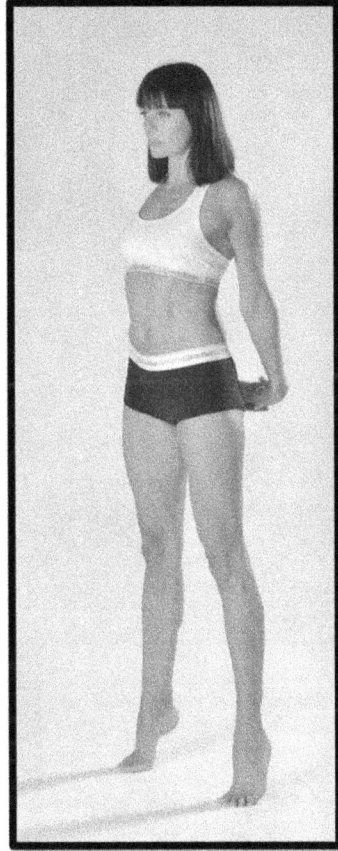

With your arms out in front of you, pull one arm toward the opposite shoulder with the other hand to stretch your shoulder. Do both arms.

Place your clasped hands behind you. Pull down as you arch your shoulders back and down to stretch your chest.

NOTE: *No need to stand on your toes. That's Inara.*

k) <u>Forearm Stretch-1</u>

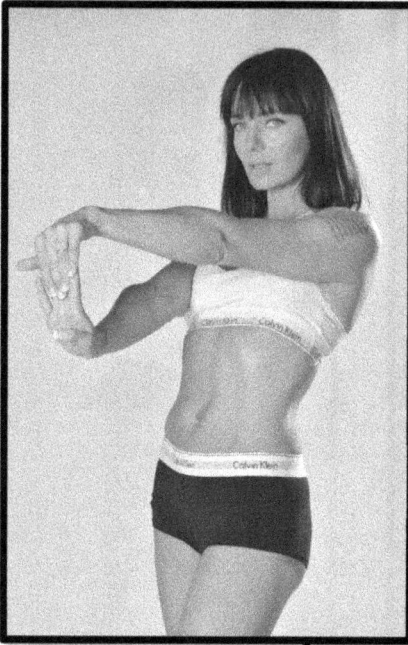

With your arms straight out, pull back on the palm-out, upturned fingers of one hand with the other hand, trying to stretch the inside of your forearms. Do both arms.

l) <u>Forearm Stretch-2</u>

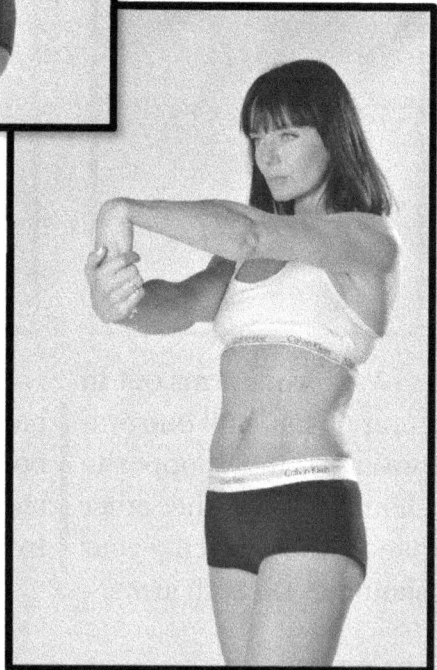

With your arms straight out, pull back on the back of the downturned fingers of one hand with the other hand, trying to stretch the outside of your forearms. Do both arms.

m) <u>Triceps Stretch</u>

Put both arms over your head, bent at the elbows. Bend one arm straight down. Grab the elbow of that arm with your other hand and pull it further down, trying to stretch the triceps of the downward arm. Do both arms.

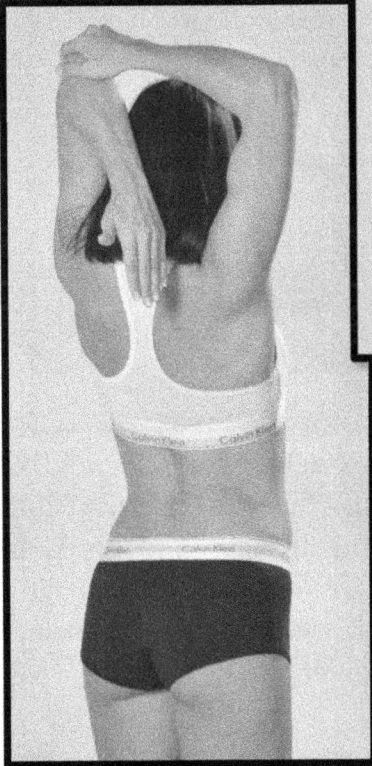

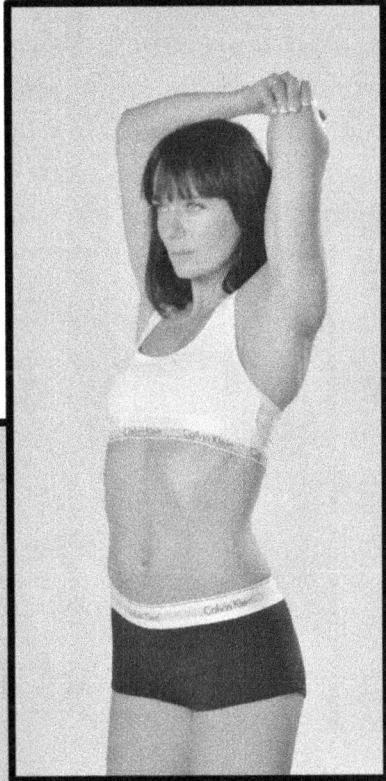

This second shot isn't really necessary, but the way we look at it... is probably the same way you're looking at it.

#7 DUO STRETCHES

Not every muscle can be worked out with a duo workout but following are a few stretching exercises that you can do with a partner, although the exercise below stretches only your imagination. Besides, it's a bit one sided. Inara has to do all the balancing.

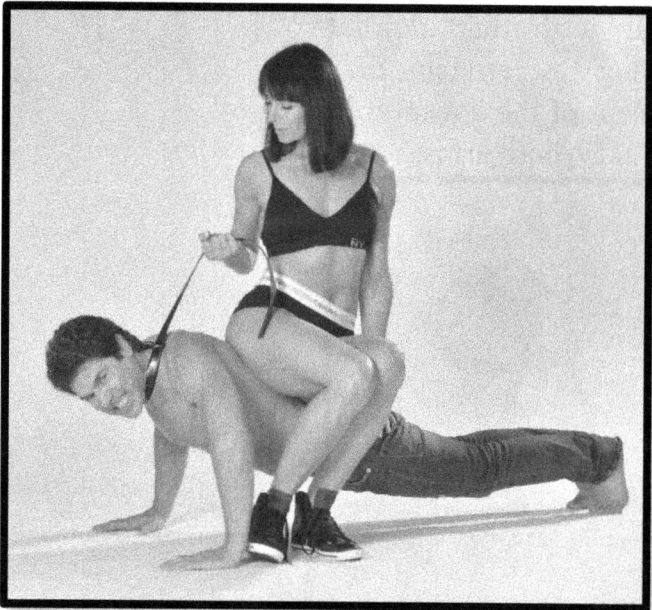

Above, Inara might be stretching her obliques, but she is mainly stretching the belt, while Billy is uncontrollably stretching his abs and his neck. Not to mention being a bit out there, this isn't a true Duo Stretch because it would be hard to switch positions. Inara would never let him do it.

WARNING: Have safe words like, "OW" or "STOP".

a) <u>Duo Hamstring Stretch</u>

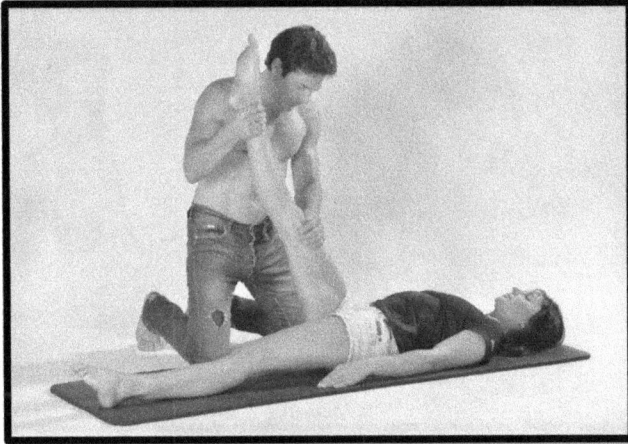

While lying face up, your partner raises one of your straight legs at a time, stretching your hamstrings.

b) <u>Duo Quad Stretch</u>

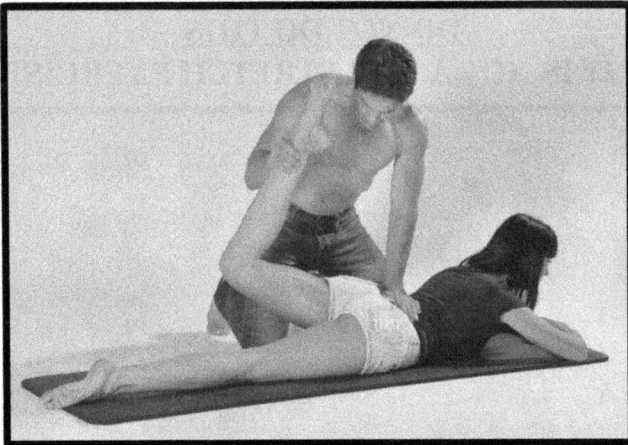

While lying face down, your partner pulls one of your bent legs back at a time, to stretch your Quads.

c) Duo Inner-Thigh/Butt Stretch

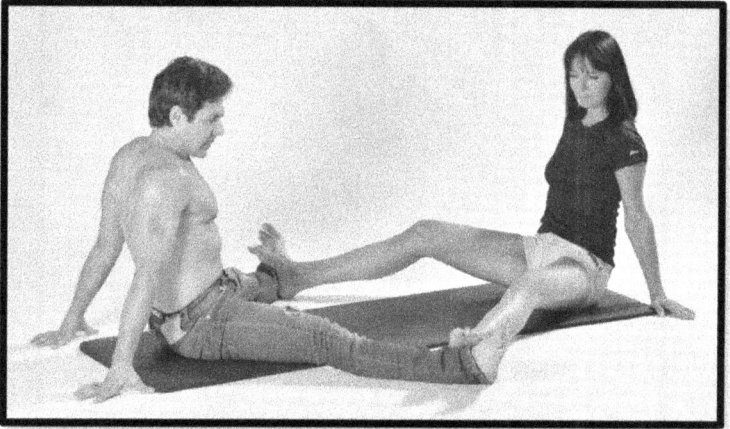

While sitting opposite each other, one person pushes out on the partner's ankles with their feet to stretch their inner-thighs and butt.

**DO NOT DO THIS –
IT IS NOT A DUO STRETCH EXERCISE**

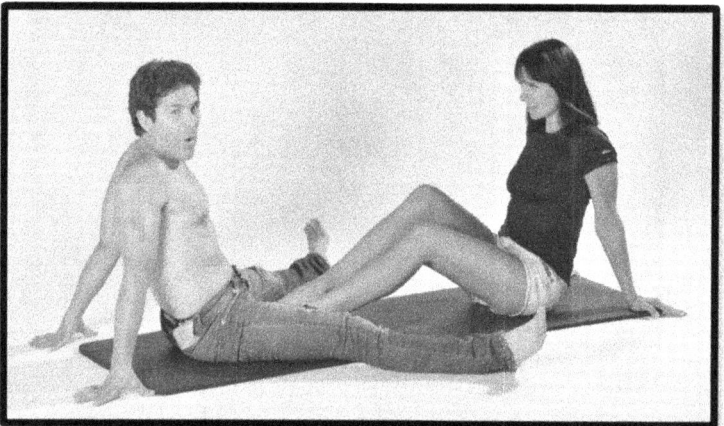

Daily/Weekly Exercise Suggestions (LEVEL II)

Just like in LEVEL I, the idea is to make exercising throughout the day a habit. So, do your best to do at least one **Xer-task** daily or several times during the week. But if you can do a series of them that's better.

Start with either an exercise of your choice or from the suggested list below. They target the large muscles of the butt and stomach and a few others that probably are not doable in public, as follows:

<u>Squats, Lunges and Backward Leg Lifts</u>

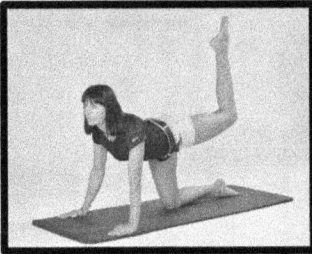

Backward Leg Lifts
(Version #1)
(S1-L II-1f)

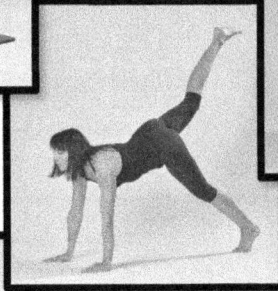

Backward
Leg Lifts
(Version #2)
(S1-L II-1f)

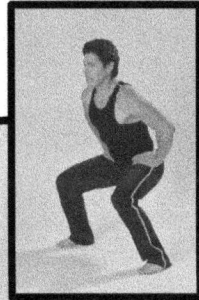

Standard
Squats
(S1-L II-1a)

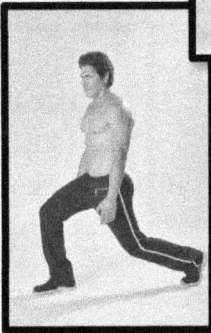

Standard Lunges (S1-L II-1d)

The Zero-Minute Workout

Various Stomach Exercises and Front Leg Lifts

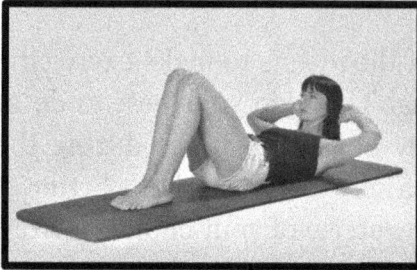

Standard
Crunch
(S1-L II-2a)

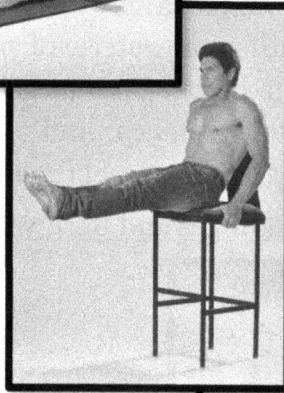

Forward
Leg Lifts
(sitting)
(Version #1)
(S1-L II-2f)

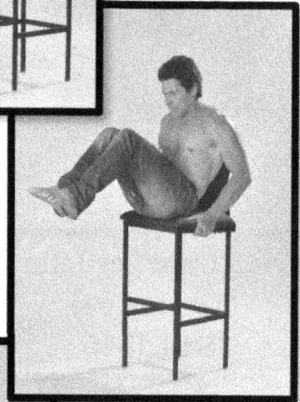

Forward
Leg Lifts
(sitting)
(Version #2)
(S1-L II-2f)

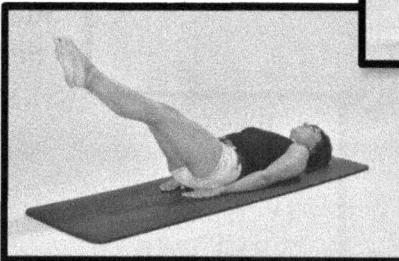

Forward Leg Lifts (lying down)
(Version #2) (S1-L II-2e)

Push-Ups

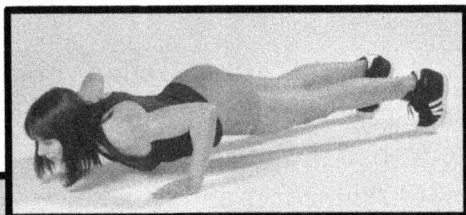

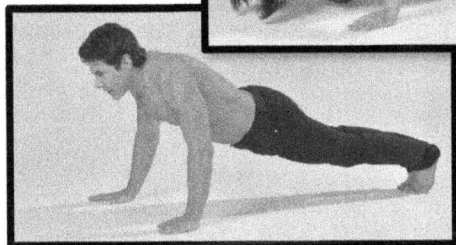

Standard Push-Ups (Version #2) (S1-L II-2a)

Standard Push-Ups (Version #1) (S1-L II-2a)

Aerobics

Curls, Lifts and Pushes

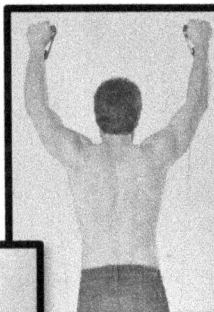

Chest "Rope Pull" (S1-L II-4f)

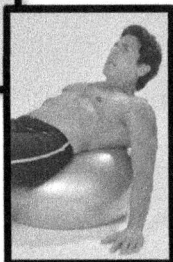

Shoulder Lift (S1-L II-4h)

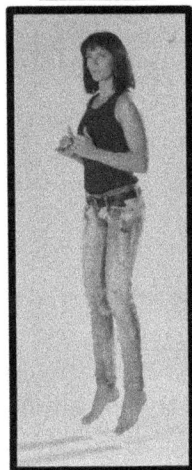

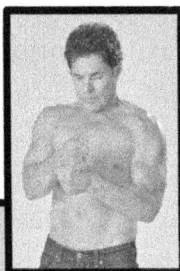

Basic Hopping (S1-L II-5a)

Freestyle Curls (S1-L II-4b)

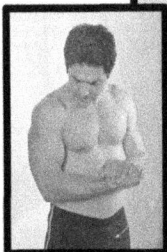

Medicine-Ball Neck Lifts (S1-L II-4j)

LEVEL III: Muscle Resistance

Like LEVEL II, this section involves primarily isokinetic exercises that may be familiar, but the variations involved may not. They generally require a little more skill, effort and resistance. Again, you may need some creative time management.

If you find that you can rearrange a block of consecutive, devoted time for exercising then you may want to consider actually doing one of the exercise routines in STAGE 2, STAGE 3 or STAGE 4 instead, or in addition. STAGE 1 has its limits, but you don't have to. By all means, if you are ready, then move on.

Suggested Accessories*:
exercise mat
elastic bands
jump rope
medicine-ball
chin-up bar/arm straps
push-up stands
two sets of free weights (i.e. 5lb/10lb; 10lb/15lb; 15lb/20lb)

*If you don't have these or don't want to get them then substitute an accessory or do an exercise that doesn't require them. As always, your progress is your choice. Exercises that don't need accessories are still going to be effective, just maybe some not to the same degree.

#1 BUTT and LEG EXERCISES

As always, when performing squats or lunges, do only those that don't cause pain in your knees. But as far as soreness goes, if you're doing things right, there isn't much way around it for almost any exercise.

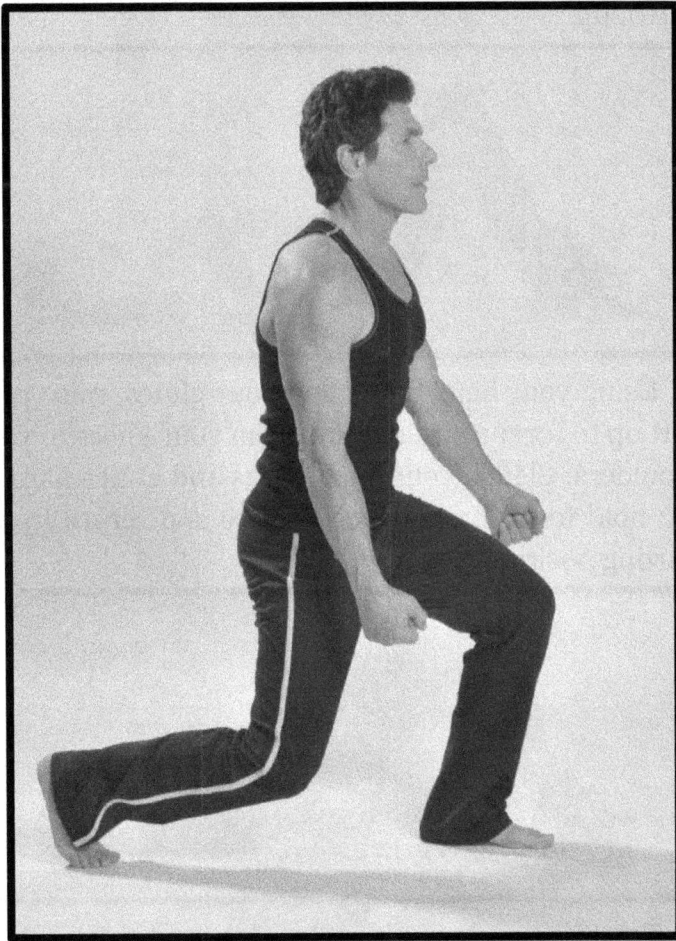

a) <u>Bridge Butt Lifts</u>

(main muscles: butt, hamstrings and quads)

Version #1: Facing upward on your back, place your feet and hands flat on the floor, with your knees drawn up.

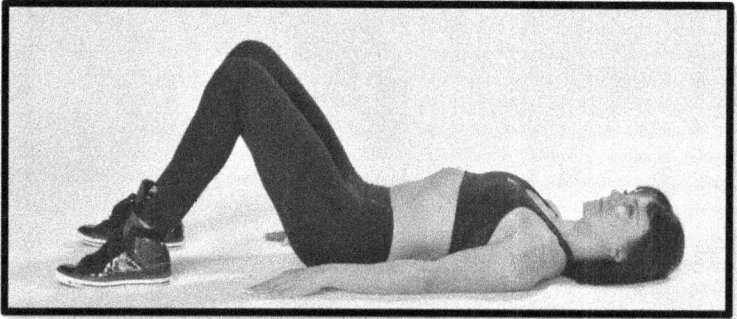

Using your hamstrings and your glutes, raise your butt up to form a straight line from your knees to your shoulders. Clench your hamstrings and glutes hard as you hold for a three-count. Release and return to the starting position.

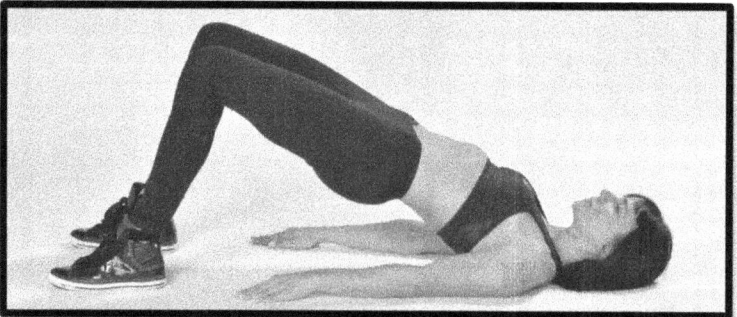

Ten to twenty reps is quite a lot. And three sets is more than good.

Version #2: This exercise starts almost the same as Version #1 except one leg is extended straight out and the other is bent with your knee up.

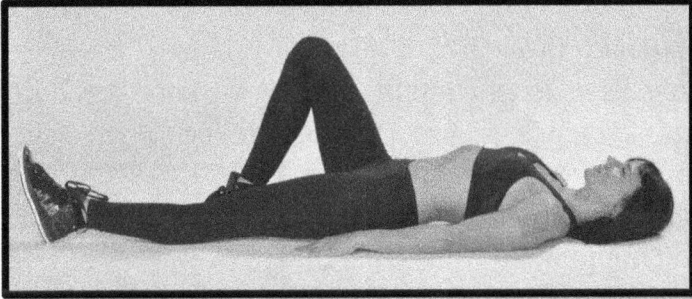

Keep one leg straight as you raise up with the other using primarily your glutes. Hold for a few seconds, then lower down to the starting position. Do this for at least five to ten reps on one leg and then the other. Repeat for three sets, whenever (and if) you can.

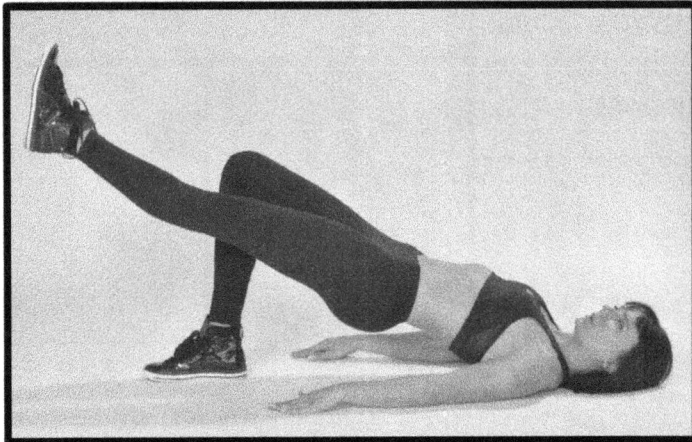

NOTE: *This version works your butt muscles the most and your hamstrings only a little.*

b) Jumping Lunges

(main muscles: quads, butt and hamstrings)

Begin these like a Standard Lunge, except this time, as soon as you lunge down with one leg, hop up and switch legs for the next lunge. Try to rely on your glutes as much as possible when lunging down and hopping up.

Continue with an equal amount on each leg for six to ten reps. Try doing three sets, (or more) with breaks. And you can do them over the course of the day if you choose.

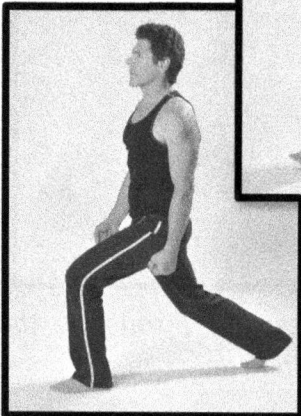

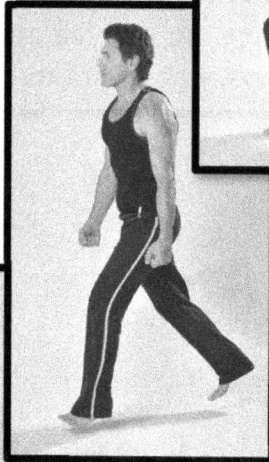

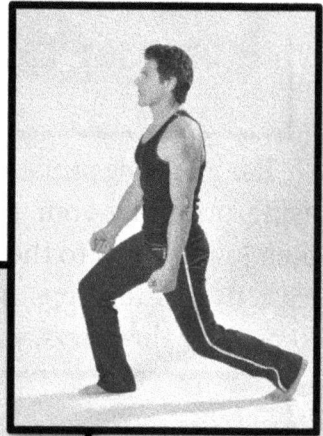

NOTE: *Unlike a Standard Lunge, your knees shouldn't go to the floor, for the sake of safety.*

c) <u>Lunge Walking</u>

(main muscles: quads, butt and hamstrings)

Version #1: Lunge Walking is exactly like it sounds: doing a lunge every step you take. With each step, on each leg, lower your back knee as far as you feel comfortable, always careful not to hit bottom.

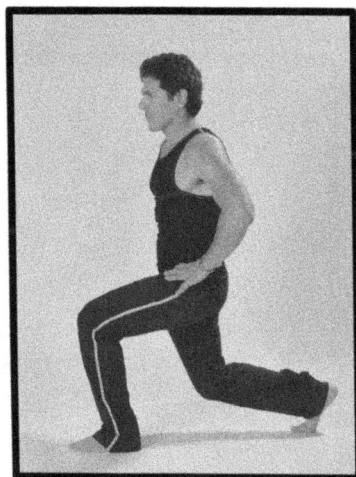

If you haven't done a lunge in a while, Lunge Walking may be a challenge. In fact the best way to do them is to set a goal – say ten to twenty steps, or a visual mark and then challenge yourself to go the distance.

Do a few sets with breaks or do them throughout the day.

Version #2: Add a leg lift after each step to increase the workout on your butt. You may not be able to do as many, but try.

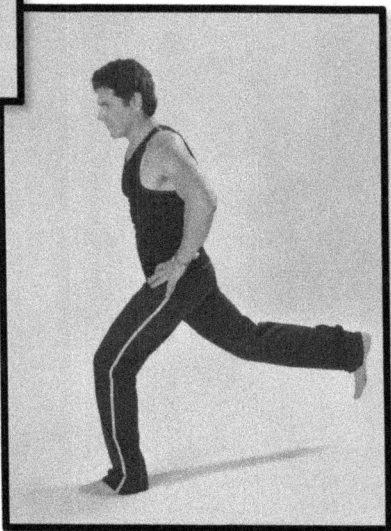

d) <u>Triple Squats</u>

(main muscles: quads, butt, hamstrings, biceps and abs)

This is a three-part set of squats.

PART I – Do ten reps of Standard Squats. Lower as far as you feel comfortable.

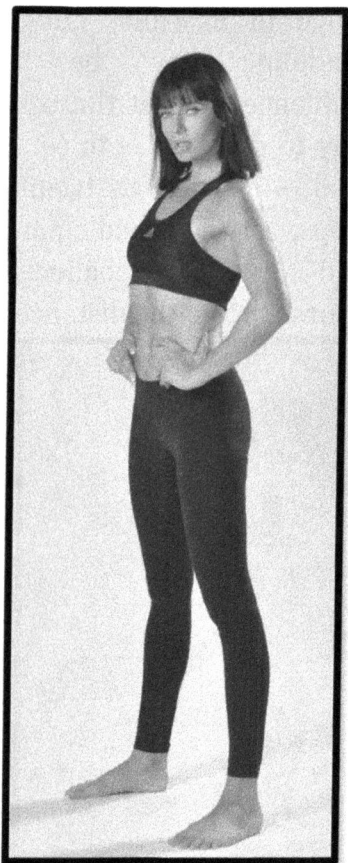

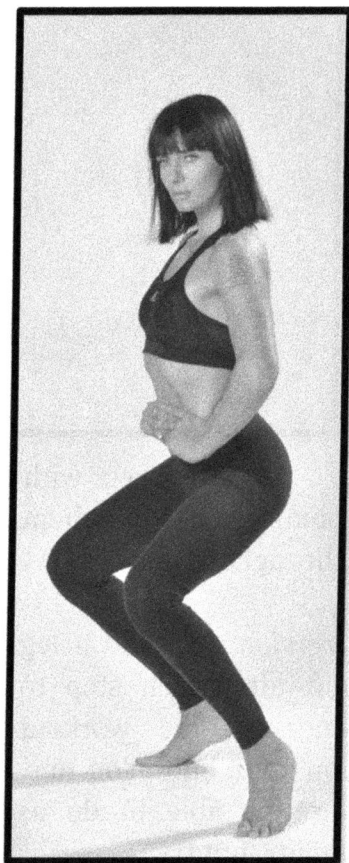

PART II – These are Standard Squats with the addition of a ten to twenty pound weight* held in your hands, for ten reps.

Start with the weight held straight down and raise it up to your chest as you lower into the squat. Return the weight to the starting position as you stand.

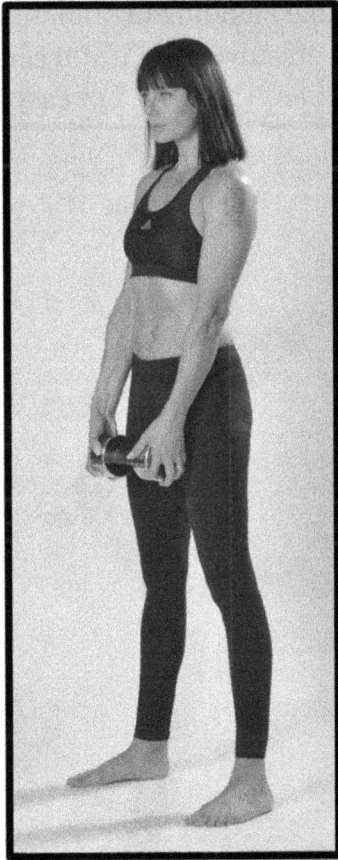

If you didn't already start to feel it after Part I, you certainly should by the end of Part II.

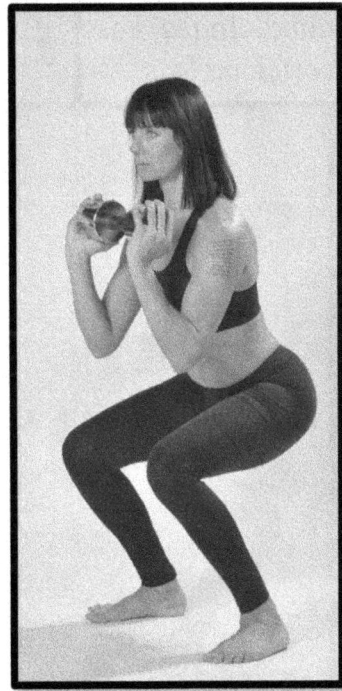

*NOTE: What you lift (i.e. dumbbells, weight plates, a sack of potatoes, etc.) and how heavy, is up to you. Just don't overdo it. You still have Part III to go.

PART III – Do what starts as a Standard Squat, but the twist is, as you stand back up, do a forward leg kick as high as you can to end the rep. Then go right back into a squat and alternate legs on each kick for a total of ten reps.

Do three sets of all three Parts (one right after the other) and you may have trouble standing or walking. They are that intense and that effective. And if you can only do one or two sets, that's fine. These are not easy.

NOTE: *Keep in mind, Inara has very long legs.*

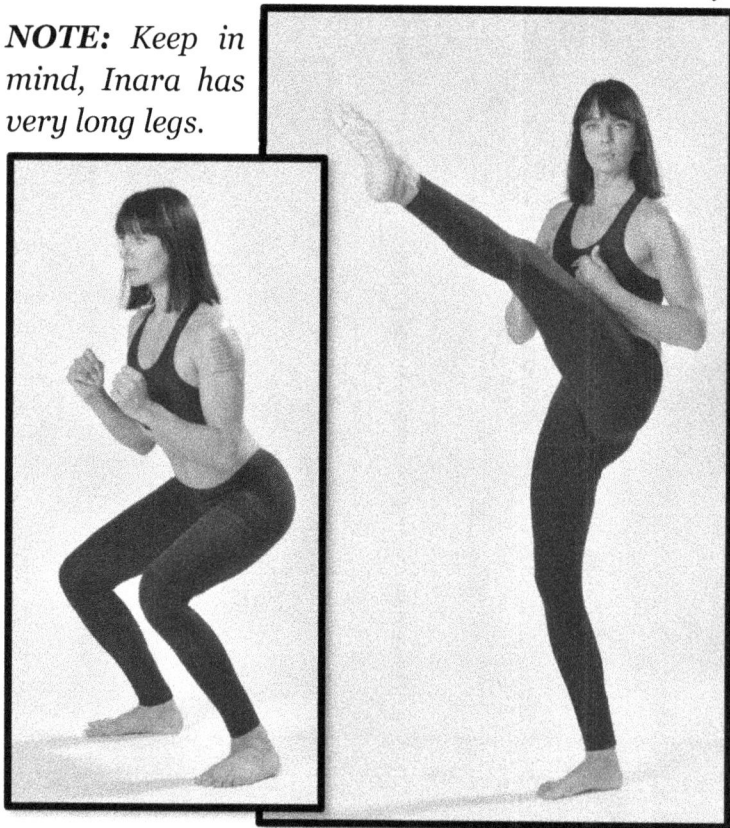

WARNING: *If you feel dizzy, STOP. Take a break.*

e) <u>Extended-Leg Floor Squat</u>

(main muscles: glutes, quads, abs and hamstrings)

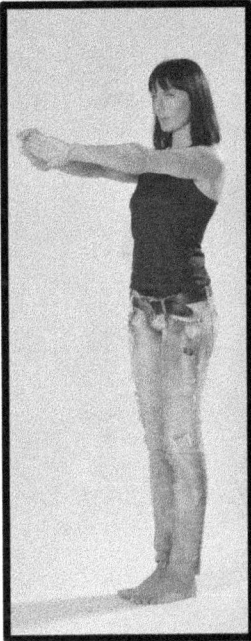

First, you should know that, THIS EXERCISE IS VERY DIFFICULT*.

With your arms straight forward, raise one leg as you slowly lower yourself to the floor. The idea here, is to get one leg as close and level to the floor as you can. Then, if you got that far, slowly raise back up the same way.

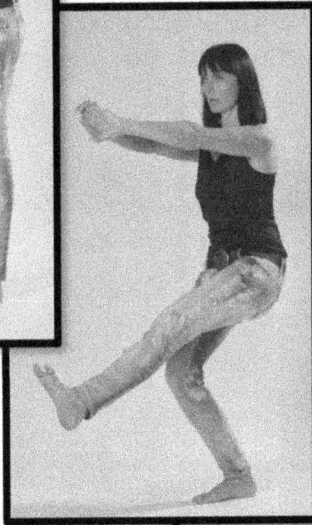

*Three reps on each leg is enough, if you can even do one. Just because Inara can do them without showing strain, that doesn't mean it's normal. It's not.

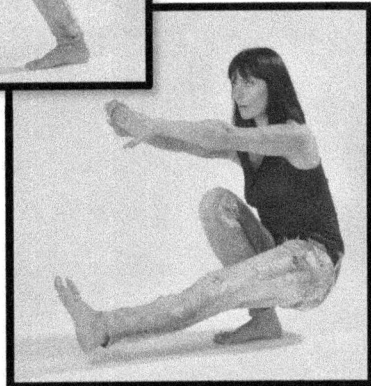

f) <u>Single-Leg Lunges (with weights)</u>

(main muscles: glutes, quads, hamstrings and biceps)

Starting with one knee raised at waist height – and with weights in hand – do these like a Standard Lunge except this time, go all the way down to the floor on one shin. Then come back up.

Alternating legs, do as many reps as you are able. And as always, if you feel pain anywhere, STOP.

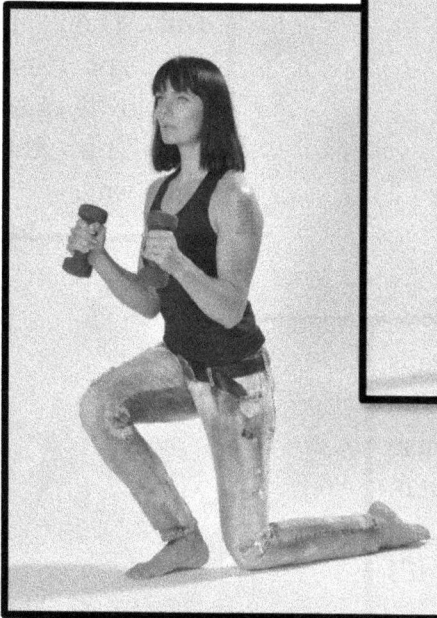

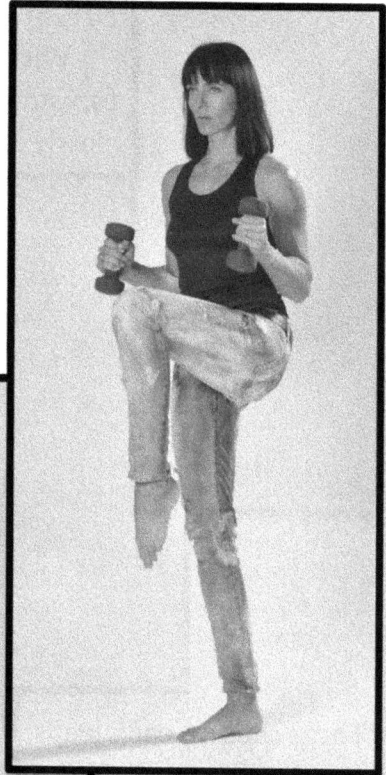

NOTE: *Weights (2-20 lbs each) will make these lunges harder but will also help your balance.*

g) <u>Sitting Hip Abductor</u>

(main muscles: glutes, thighs)

Like the LEVEL I Clench, this exercise works your glutes and outer thighs where they connect to your hips. And depending on the band strength used, it could be either a LEVEL II or a LEVEL III exercise. For LEVEL III we suggest using a strong elastic band.

While sitting, with your legs together, place a band around your thighs at the knees. Engage your glutes as you push out against the band and hold for five seconds at least. Slowly return to the start and repeat for 50-100 reps (broken into groups you can handle).

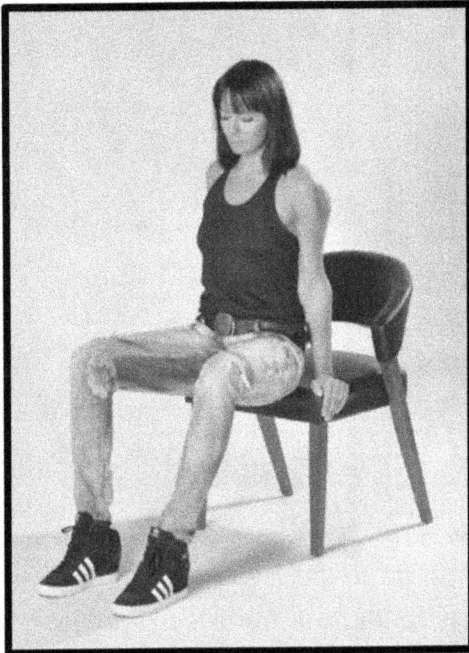

The idea is to exhaust your butt. And if you're not, then visualize and try again.

HINT: raise off your butt for an increased burn.

LEVEL I:
#1 THE BUTT –
g) Sitting Hip Abductor Clench, offers a non-moving version.

h) <u>Calves Lift</u>

(main muscles: calves)

While standing, place your feet parallel to each other with one foot twelve inches in front of the other. With a weight (of your choice) in each hand, rise up on your toes, tensing your calves. Hold and lower back down. Do ten lifts. Switch the position of your feet for ten more. Do at least three sets.

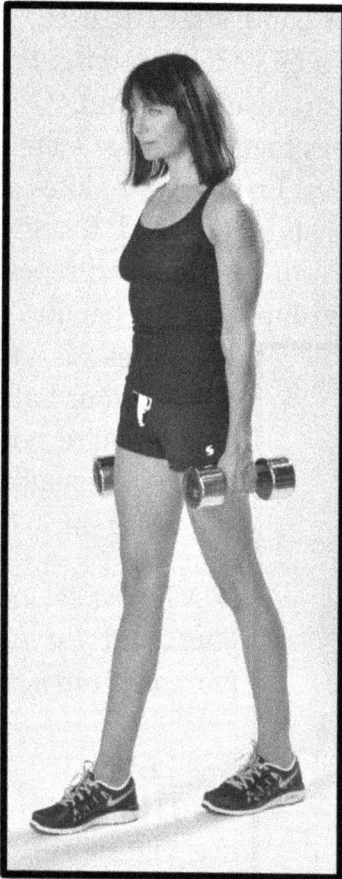

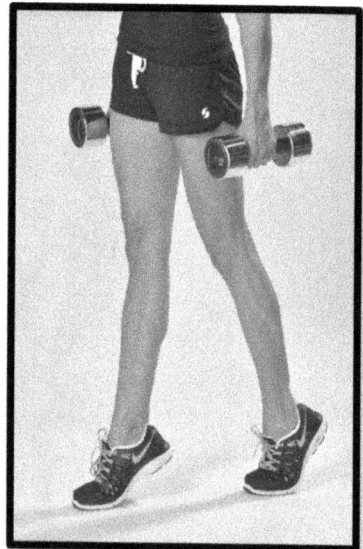

NOTE: *If you don't have access to any kind of weights, simply raise up without them. Just do more.*

#2 VARIOUS STOMACH EXERCISES

These exercises are more intense than those in the Intermediate section but they are only effective if you can do them. There's no shame if you're not ready yet.

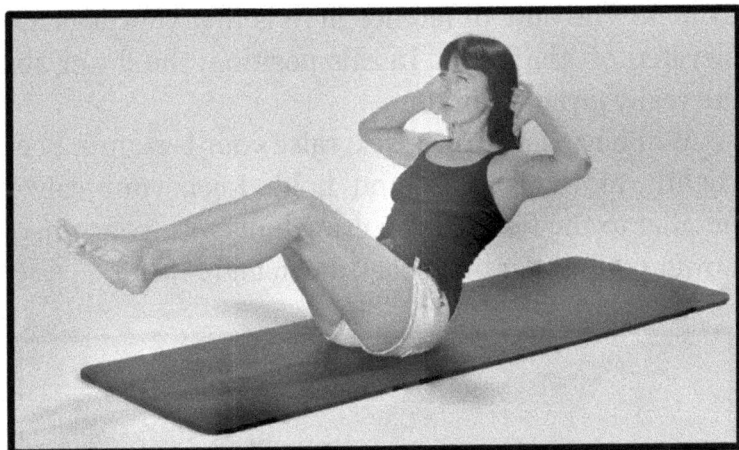

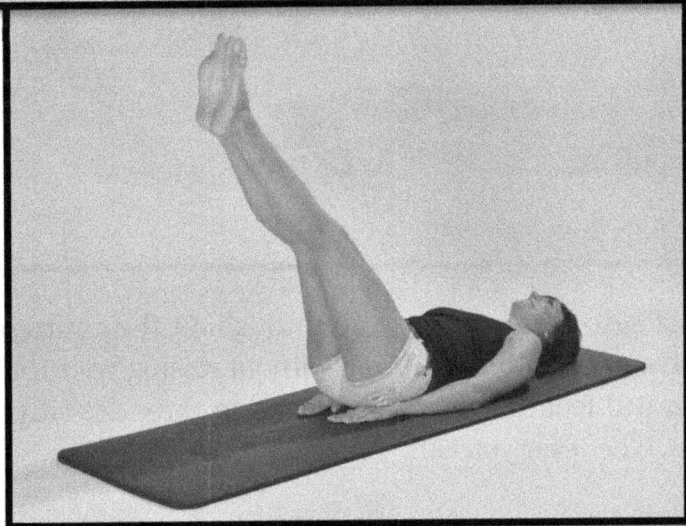

a) <u>Elevated Crunch</u>

(main muscles: lower abs and quads)

This is performed exactly like the Standard Crunch. The only difference here is that your legs are elevated off the floor. In this position, the lower abs are really given a workout.

While lying on your back, raise your legs up – bent slightly at the knee – and hold. Keep your calves parallel to the floor as you crunch up with your torso. Lower your upper body back down and repeat.

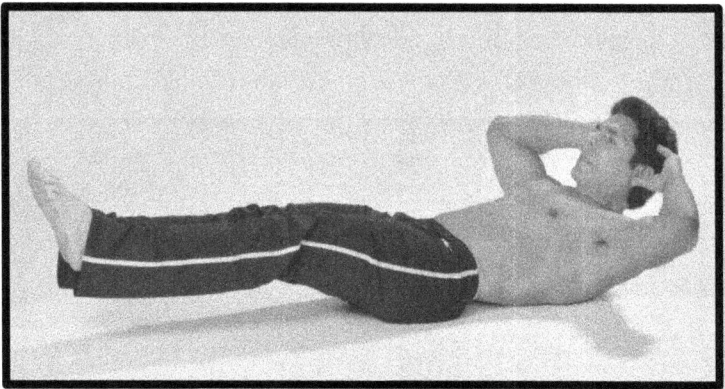

Try to hold your legs up throughout the entire set of twenty to fifty reps. Even without raising your torso you will feel this one. And again, do three sets if you can, whenever you can.

b) Elevated Crunch (with a twist)

(main muscles: quads, obliques and lower abs)

This exercise is done just like the Elevated Crunch but with an added twist.

As you raise your torso twist one elbow to the opposite side. Make sure you keep your legs elevated the whole time.

Challenge yourself to do as many reps as you can over ten, working both sides equally. And do three sets if you're able, even if it takes you the rest of the day.

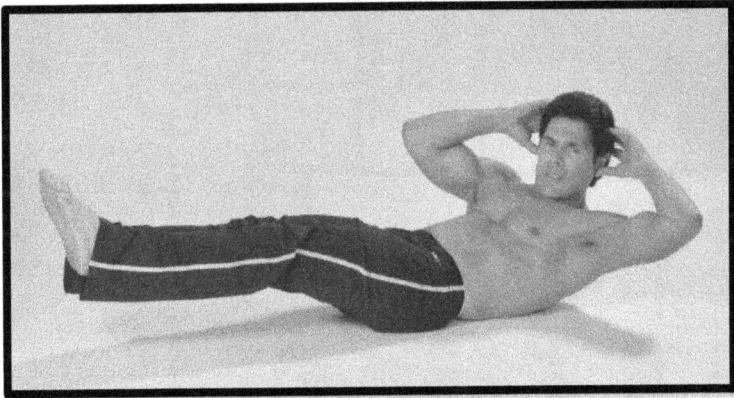

In this position, not only will your obliques be worked but your core balance will also be utilized.

NOTE: Although Billy is not using any kind of a cushion for his back, we still recommend that you do. Just because Billy is too cool for a mat doesn't mean that you should try it too. But it's your choice.

c) Elevated Twisting Crunch (with weight)

(main muscles: obliques and lower abs)

These are performed from the full-crunch position of an Elevated Crunch, with the addition of a weight, such as a dumbbell held in both hands (a large bag of potatoes might work in a pinch).

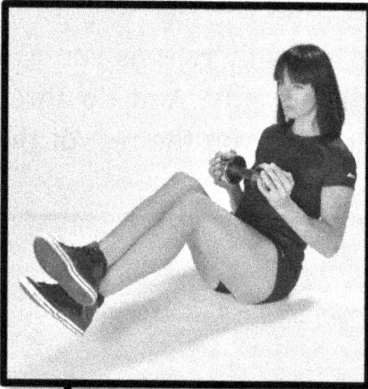

Grip the weight firmly as you forcefully swing it from side to side, with your bent legs swinging slightly to the opposite side for balance. Move the weight as far to each side as you can and feel comfortable in so doing.

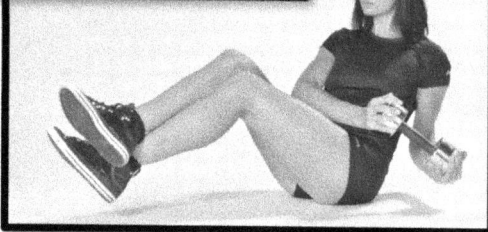

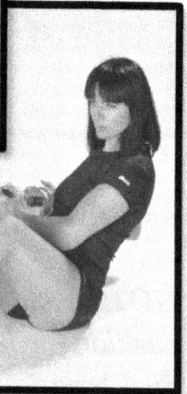

Try for ten complete, side-to-side reps, rest and go for three sets.

NOTE: *Crossing your legs helps your balance as you swing the weight, working your core.*

d) <u>Folding Crunch</u>

(main muscles: abs and quads)

Just getting to the starting position is an exercise, with this. Your abs and thighs are constantly tensed.

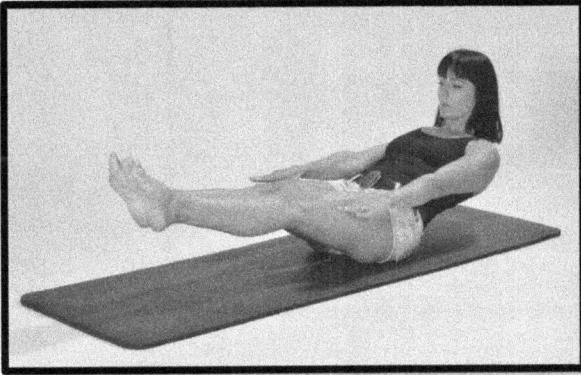

In the shape of a low "V" – your arms and legs stretched forward; your torso and head raised up – fold your legs to your chest and bring your chest up to meet them. Return to the starting position and do twenty to thirty reps for three sets.

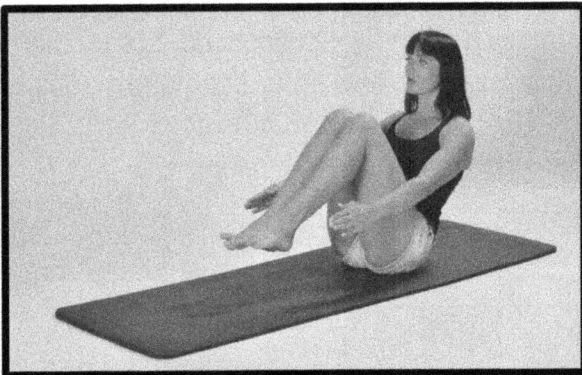

e) <u>Scissor Leg Lifts Combo</u>

(main muscles: lower abs and thighs)

PART I – With your hands under your hips, start with your legs straight out at a 45 degree angle or higher to

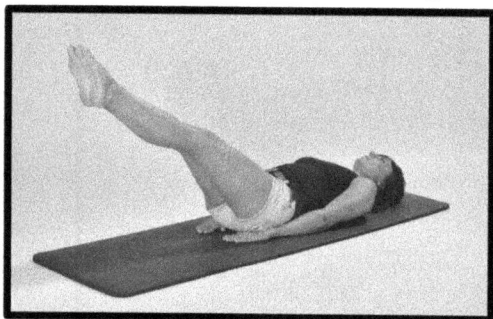

the floor. Lower them to just off the floor (as below). Hold, then raise them back up. Hold and repeat for ten reps.

Now, WITHOUT STOPPING...

PART II – Start with your feet together and hovering just above the floor.

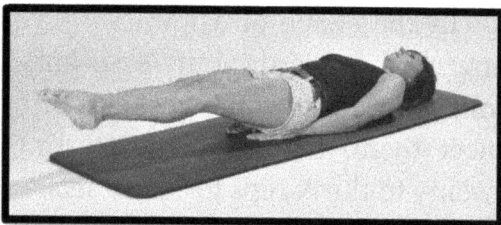

Briefly spread your legs wide and hold. Then bring them back together and hold, keeping them raised for ten reps. Rest and do two more sets of Part I and II.

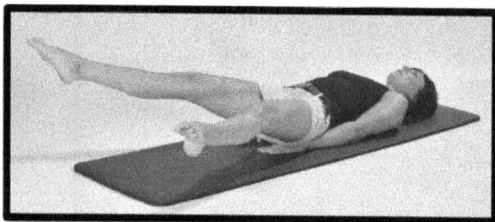

NOTE: If you can only do one Part at a time, then just do that one.

f) <u>Medicine-Ball Crunch</u>

(main muscles: stomach)

Start by lying on a medicine-ball at the middle of your back. With your feet flat on the floor and your hands by your sides (or at your head), raise your torso up to crunch your abs, then return. Go for twenty to

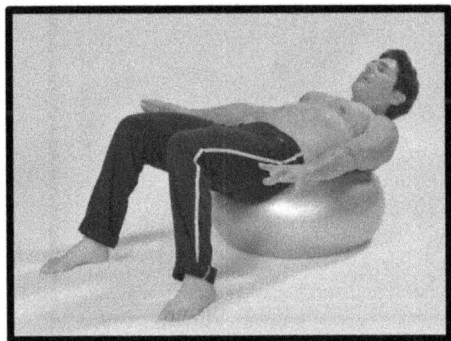

forty reps and three sets. And if you can do more, do it.

Doing crunches on a medicine-ball will save your back from unnecessary strain. And trying to keep your balance will additionally work your obliques*.

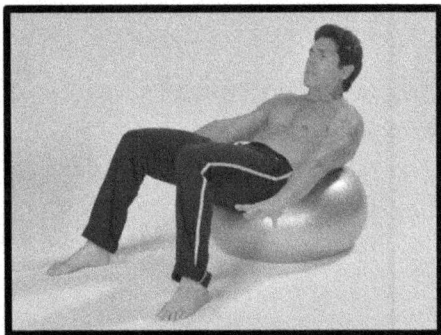

*NOTE: For a more targeted workout on your obliques, turn slightly to the sides as you sit up.

g) <u>Medicine-Ball Leg Rolls</u>

(main muscles: stomach and shoulders)

Start from a push-up position, with your legs straight and your shins resting on a medicine-ball.

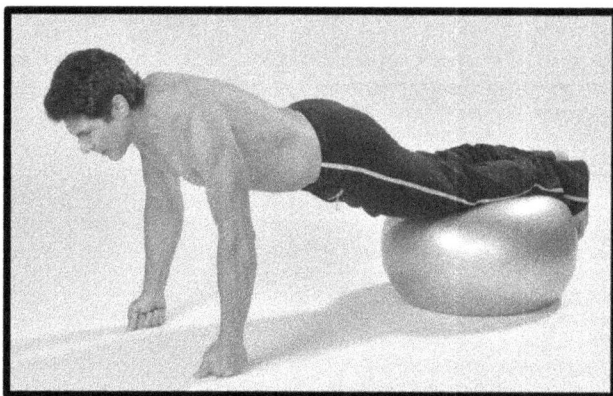

Roll your feet as far forward as possible, hold, roll your feet back and hold. Do this for as long as you can in one session. Then do it again when you're able.

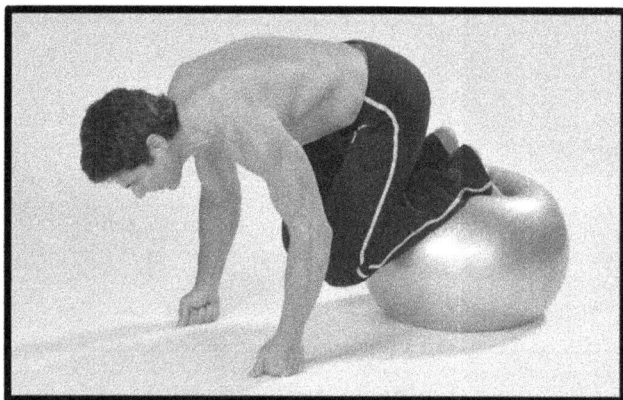

NOTE: *Using your knuckles is up to you, not Billy.*

#3 PUSH-UPS

The push-ups here are a little more difficult than in the Intermediate section. So, if you can't do them, don't worry about it. As with all the exercises, do only what you can, without strain or stress.

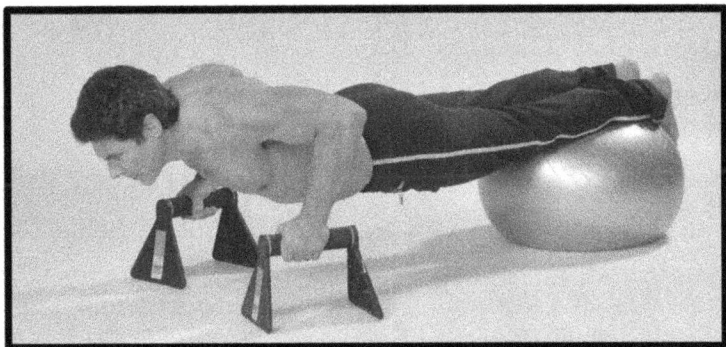

NOTE: *Push-Up stands, like those Billy's using above and below are not mandatory, but they allow for an extra stretch of your chest, shoulders and triceps as you lower yourself to the floor. More importantly, they put much less stress on your wrists, forming a more natural alignment of your arms to your hands and they can be placed in a variety of positions.*

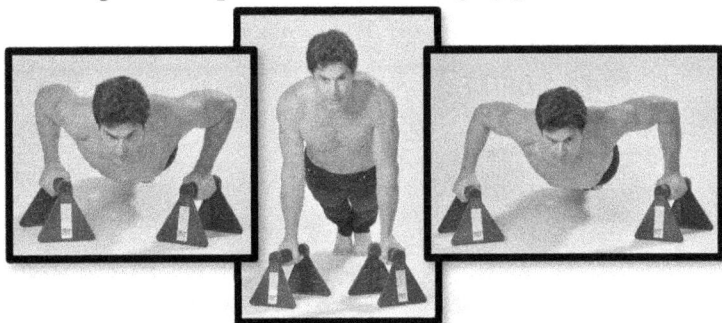

a) <u>Advanced Push-Ups</u>

(Main muscles: triceps, pecs and shoulders)

Version #1: Do these with your hands about six inches apart and your feet together. They engage your triceps much more than Standard Push-Ups and they also work your balance. Try for a cumulative total of ten to twenty or more, spread out over the day if needed.

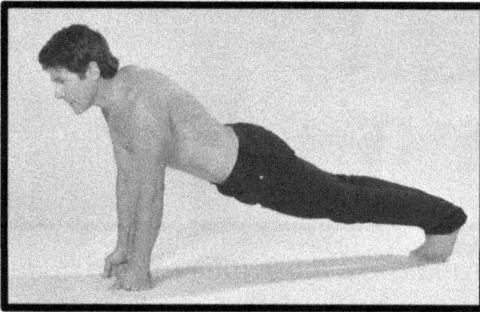

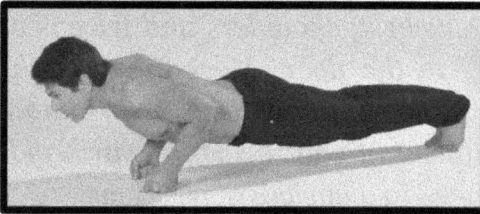

NOTE: *<u>Using your knuckles is optional.</u> Billy does them this way in place of using his Push-Up stands – no wrist stress. But if you do, we suggest using a softer surface than the floor.*

Version #2: Shaping a diamond with your hands helps work your shoulders more.

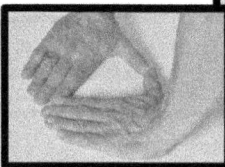

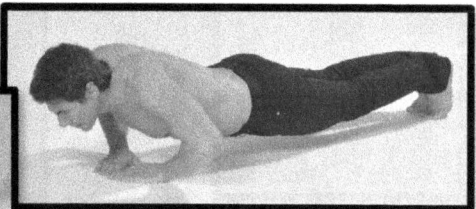

Again, ten to twenty is very good.

b) Decline Push-Ups

(main muscles: shoulders, chest and triceps)

   Start with your feet elevated on a chair, or similar object, holding your torso up with your hands under your chest. Try doing ten reps, for three sets.

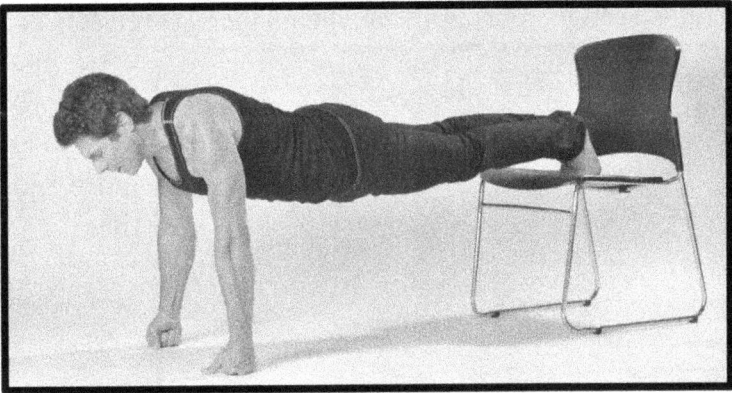

   Again, the more your hands are together, the more your triceps are worked; the wider they are apart, the more your shoulders and chest are worked.

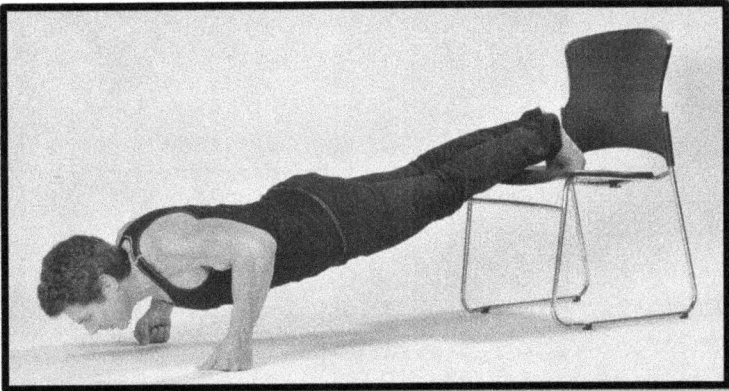

NOTE: *Knuckles/Push-Up Stands ease wrist stress.*

c) <u>Push-Ups (with Leg Lifts)</u>

(main muscles: triceps, chest, butt, shoulders and abs)

This is performed like a standard push-up, but with one leg raised back and high. Do one leg, then the other without stopping, really clenching your glutes. Ten or more reps on each leg, for three sets is a good goal. But if you can do more, do them.

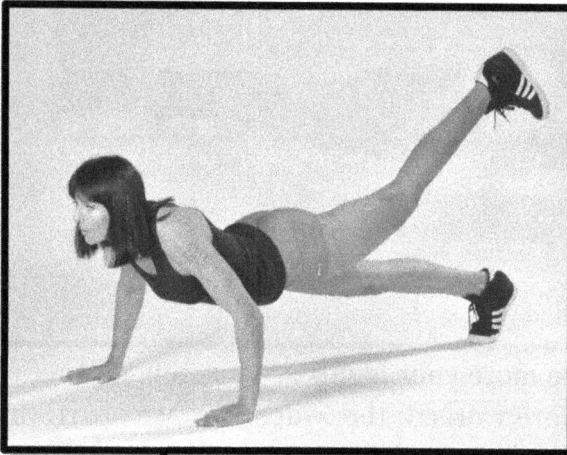

Unlike Billy, Inara is not about to use her knuckles to do Push-Ups.

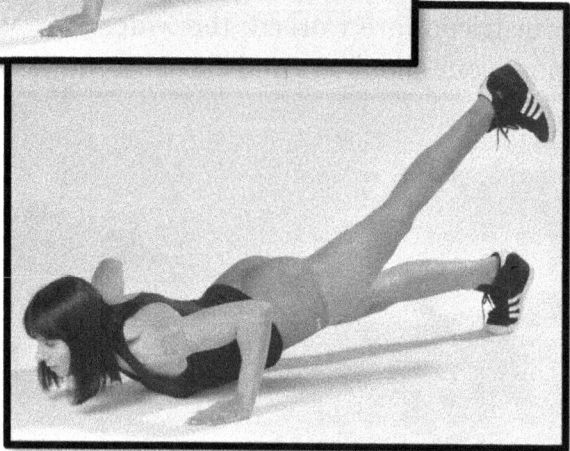

NOTE: *Push-Up Stands aren't needed, but they help.*

d) <u>Leg Crunch Push-Ups</u>

(main muscles: triceps, chest, shoulders and stomach)

Version #1: Start like a Standard Push-Up, but instead of lowering down, pivot forward at the hips, bringing one leg out to the side toward your arms, keeping that shin level with the floor.

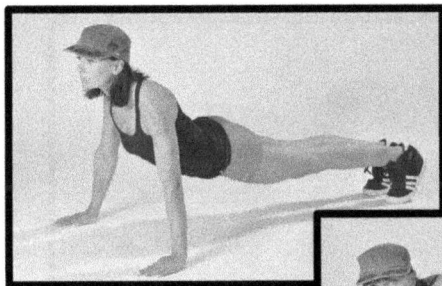

Alternate legs for ten reps total.

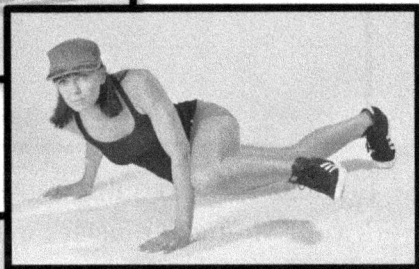

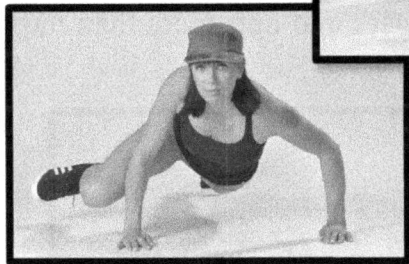

It won't be easy, but try for three sets.

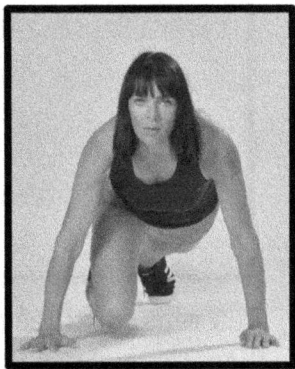

Version #2: This version is easier. Bring one leg at a time straight forward as far as you can, keeping that shin level with the floor. Alternate legs for three sets of ten reps.

Step Things Up: Do both versions one after the other.

e) <u>Medicine-Ball Push-Ups</u>

(main muscles: triceps, shoulders, abs and butt)

This exercise is performed like the Decline Push-Ups, using a medicine-ball instead of a chair.

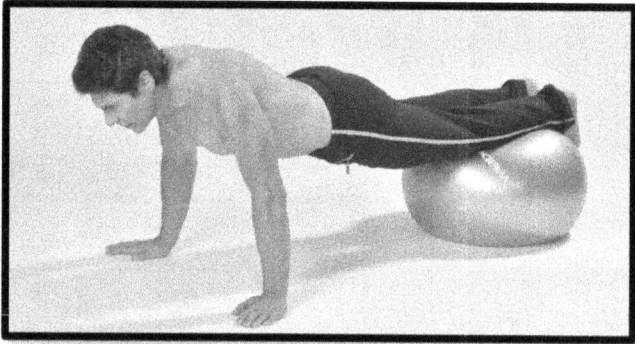

Because these require a great deal of balance they work your stomach muscles and butt more than most other push-ups.

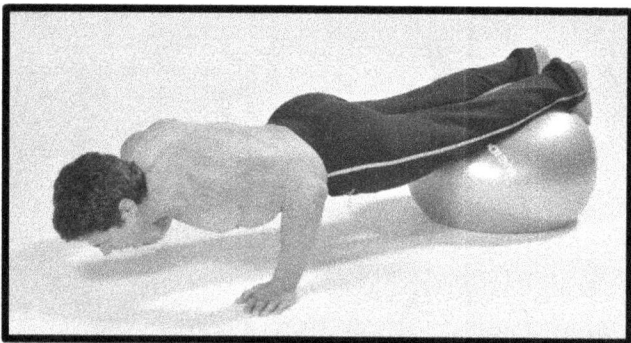

Ten reps for three sets is good even if you have to do them throughout the day.

#4 UPPER BODY

The Upper Body is probably the part of us that's most visible. That's not to say it's the most important, but it is an area that is affected quickest by exercise. Especially if you throw in some weights.

We think you'll agree, strong biceps, a toned stomach and great pecs are pretty darn good assets.

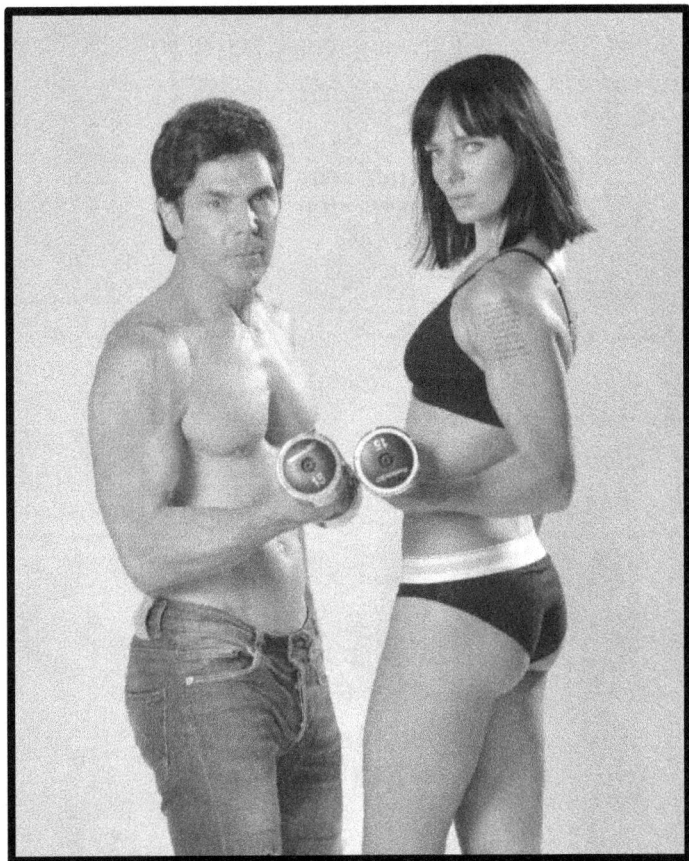

(Though a firm butt and nice legs aren't bad either.)

a) <u>Curls</u>

(main muscles: biceps)

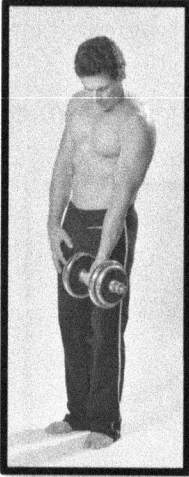

PART I – Using your choice of free weights*, extend your arms down to your sides. Curl one arm up to between your waist and chest for seven to ten reps. Repeat with your other arm.

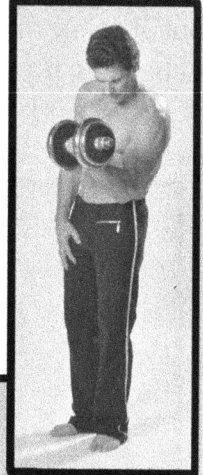

NOTE: *If you curl with both arms at a time, it won't isolate the biceps as well as using just one arm.*

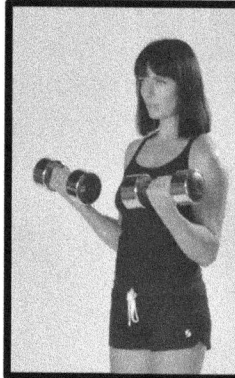

*Choose a weight that gives good resistance not strain.

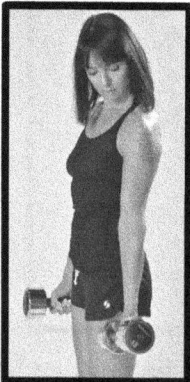

PART II – Curl your arm all the way up to your chest for seven to ten more reps. Repeat with your other arm.

Take a break and do two more sets of both Parts, for both arms.

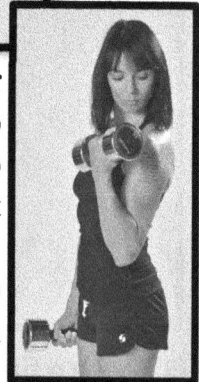

b) <u>Medicine-Ball Chest Press</u>

(main muscles: pecs)

Lay on a medicine-ball at the middle of your back, with a dumbbell in each hand (your choice of weight), your feet flat on the floor and your bent elbows level with your chest. Now, balancing with your feet,

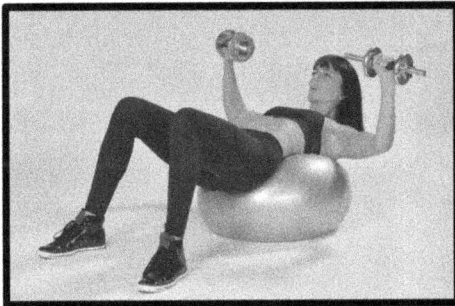

slowly press up, extending your arms straight and slowly return. Try to raise your arms steady and equally, for three sets of ten reps each.

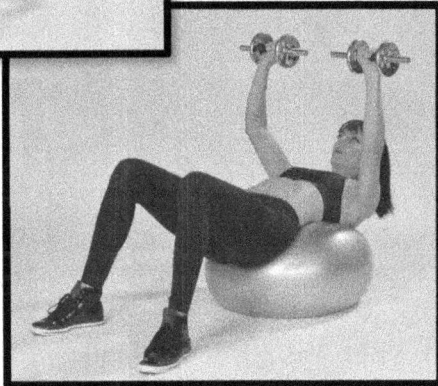

The medicine-ball works like a weight bench, with an added benefit to your core as you balance.

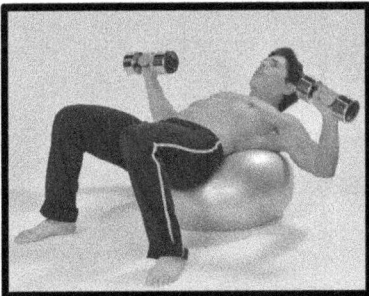

NOTE: *For an extra pecs stretch, dip your elbows as low as you can before pressing up, like Billy.*

c) <u>Full-Range Curl, Push, Press and Pull</u>

(main muscles: biceps, shoulders and lats)

Part I – Start on your knees (or standing), with one weight held in both hands and arms extended fully down, do a biceps curl up to your chest.

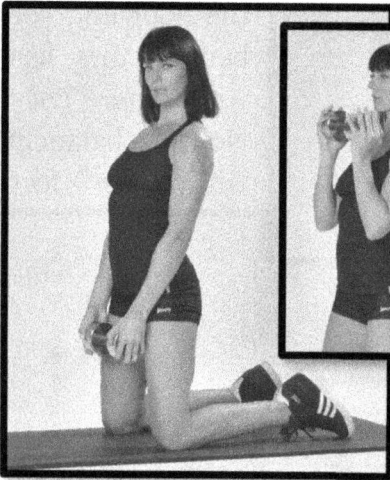

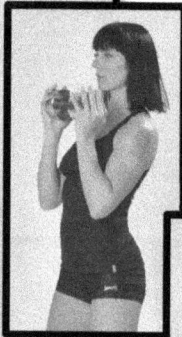

Part II – Push the weight straight out at your shoulders and hold for a beat.

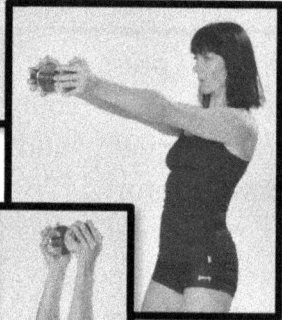

Part III – Swing your hands straight up over your head and bend them all the way back to your shoulders.

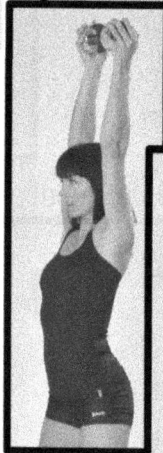

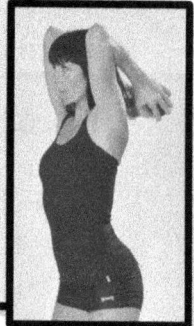

Part IV – Return your arms over your head for a triceps pull and keeping your arms straight, slowly lower them back to the start position.

Take your time doing three sets of ten full reps.

d) <u>Shoulder Press</u>

(main muscles: shoulders)

Holding weights in your hands* (turned to the side), with your elbows bent at shoulder level, raise your arms, extending them fully into the air.

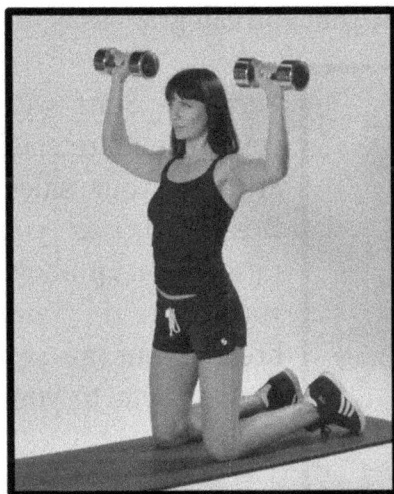

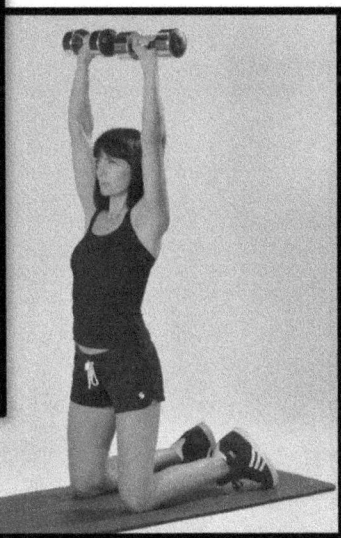

*standing or kneeling

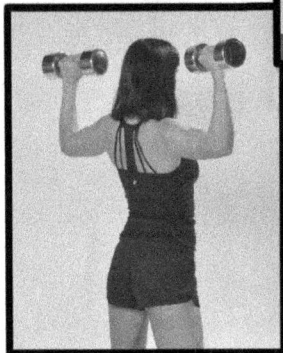

Lower the weights back to the start and repeat for the usual ten reps and three sets.

(We thought you might like a different perspective.)

WARNING: If you feel twinges anywhere, STOP.

e) Shoulder Swings (with weights)*

(main muscles: shoulders)

This three-part exercise is quite effective for the shoulders and upper arms. Use a light weight (no more than 5 pounds) – one that you can grip easily.

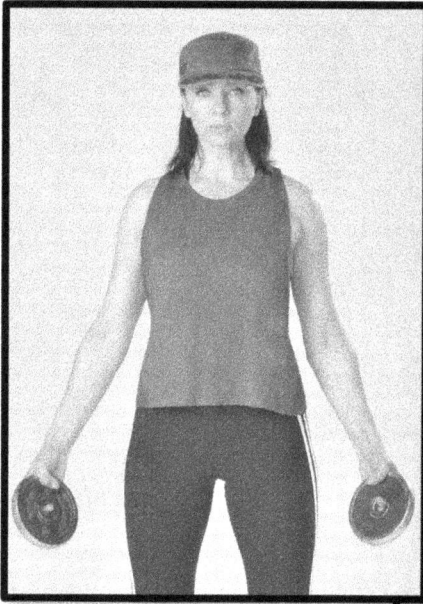

Part I – Start with your outstretched arms at your sides. Breathe in as you raise them up above your head and breathe out as you return them to your sides.

Do continuous, smooth motions for ten reps. Move on to Part II and Part III pausing between. Repeat for three sets total.

*all pictures taken 2017

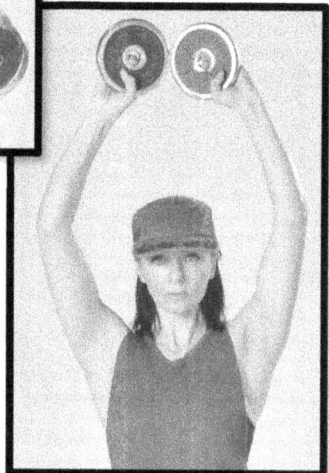

Part II – With your arms extended out to your sides, keep them level and straight as you bring them forward until the weights come together. Do three reps, pause and move on to Part III.

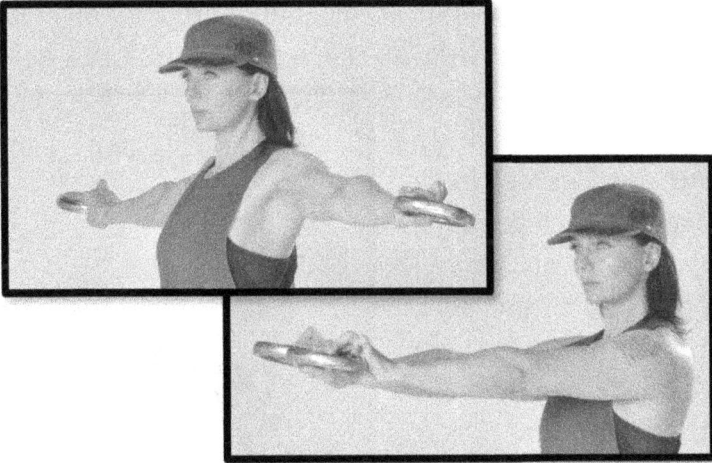

Part III – With your arms out and up at your sides, at 90 degree angles, pivot both arms down parallel to your shoulders and return for ten reps.

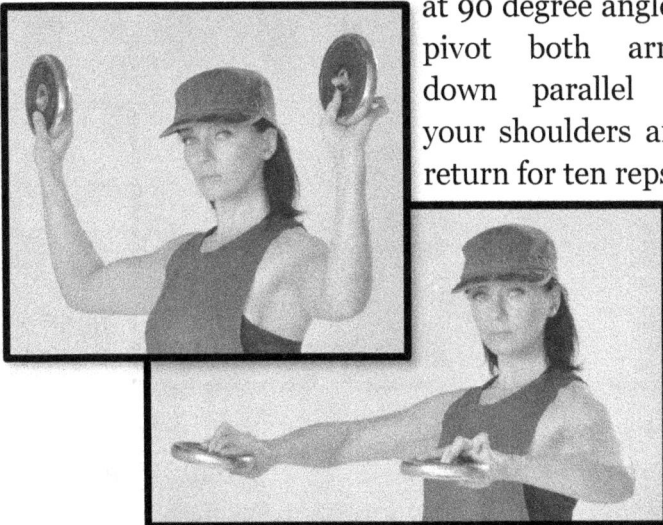

f) Backward Fly

(main muscles: shoulders)

With a light weight in each hand, crouch down and bend forward a little at the waist; your arms bent slightly at the elbows. Force your arms up and backwards in a reverse bench press.

If you can do ten reps for three sets, great. Otherwise, do what you can without straining and rest between sets.

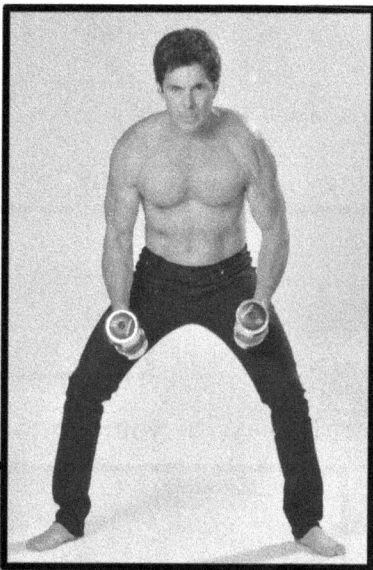

NOTE: *Your torso will move forward as your arms go back.*

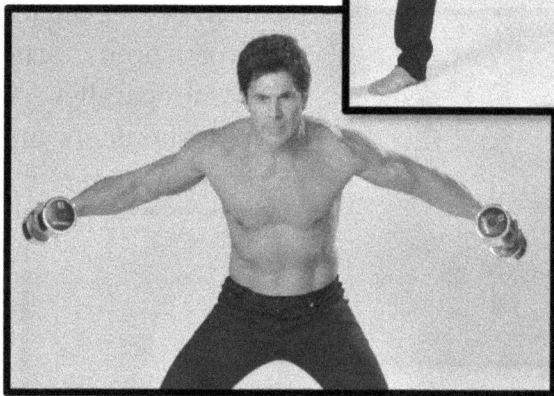

WARNING: *If you feel twinges in your shoulders, neck or arms, STOP. Take a break, use a lighter weight and try again later.*

g) <u>Lats Pull</u>

(main muscles: lats)

With a weight in one hand, rest your opposite knee on a chair, steadying yourself with your other hand. Fully extend the weighted hand all the way down.

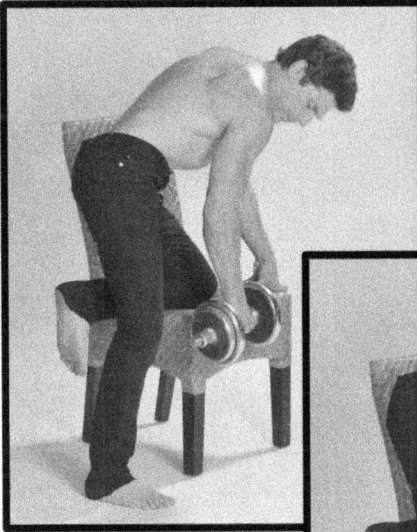

Pull the weight up toward your chest, using your lats. Lower the weight all the way down and repeat for ten reps.

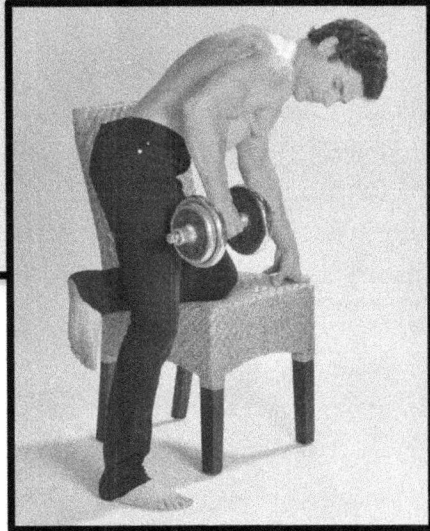

Switch positions and do the same with your other arm, for a total of three sets.

NOTE: *This is quite a strong muscle so you should be able to use a heavier weight than usual. Just don't overdo it.*

h) <u>Lunge Lats Pull</u>

(main muscles: lats and glutes)

With a weight of your choice in each hand, extend one leg far out to the side. Step slightly forward with your other leg and squat into a semi-lunge position – arms straight down – working the glutes of your bent leg.

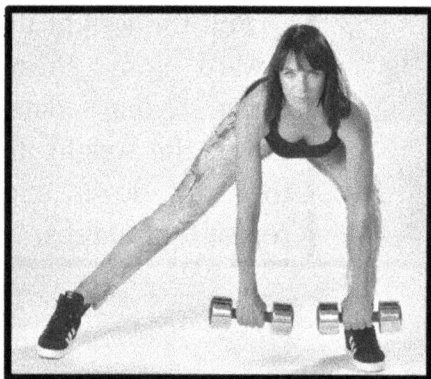

Using your lats, pull the weights to your chest, keeping your chin up.

After five reps, switch leg positions and do five more for three sets total.

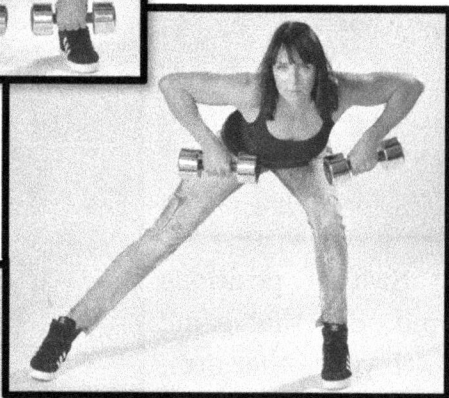

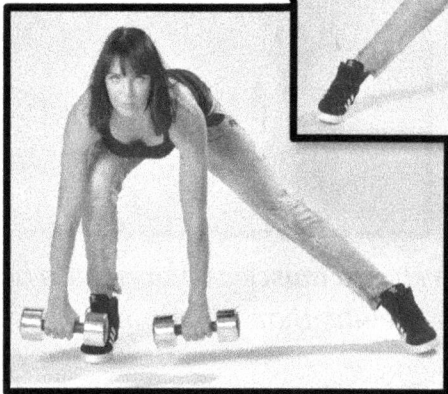

NOTE: *The weights you use should not be as heavy as for a normal Lats Pull.*

i) <u>Forearm Lifts</u>

(main muscles: forearms)

These are like curls for your forearms. While holding a dumbbell in one hand, with your hand turned away from your thighs, bend your wrist up.

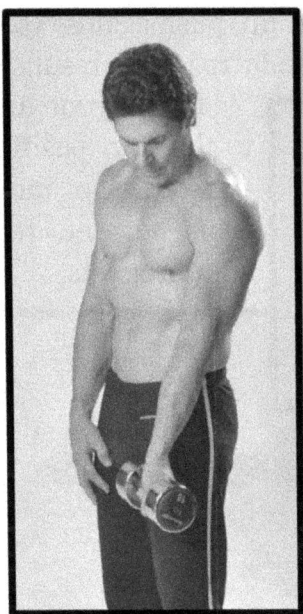

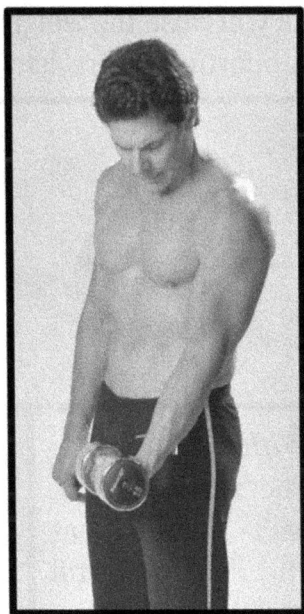

How heavy a weight you are using will determine how many reps you should do. Let that be your judge. And like always, don't go overboard using a too-heavy weight.

About ten reps or so on each arm should be enough. Take a break or do another exercise before you do a couple more sets.

j) <u>Triceps Press</u> (w/weight)*

(main muscles: triceps)

With support: While lying on a flat surface and your choice of weight in one hand, bend that arm at a 90 degree angle, with your forearm parallel to your body. As you raise the weight straight up, push against your supporting and resisting hand to increase the results.

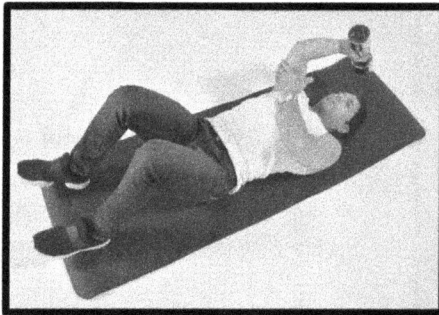

Lower your arm to the start position and do the move again for ten reps and three sets.

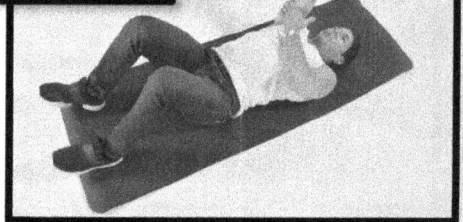

Without support: The version below isn't quite as effective, but it still works very well.

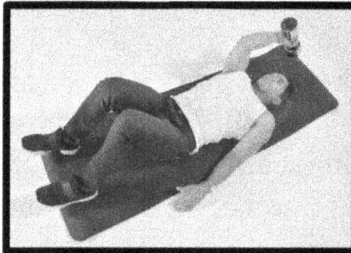

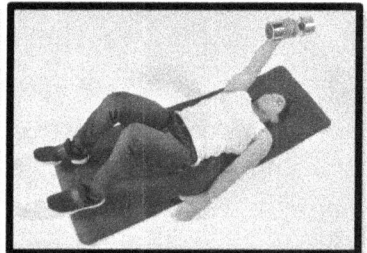

*pictures taken 2017

#5 CHIN-UP BAR EXERCISES

Many people may find it difficult to perform pull-ups and chin-ups. They are not an easy exercise. So if you can only do one or two, don't worry. If you keep at it you'll get better. But if this exercise seems like too much, then there is no need to kill yourself trying.

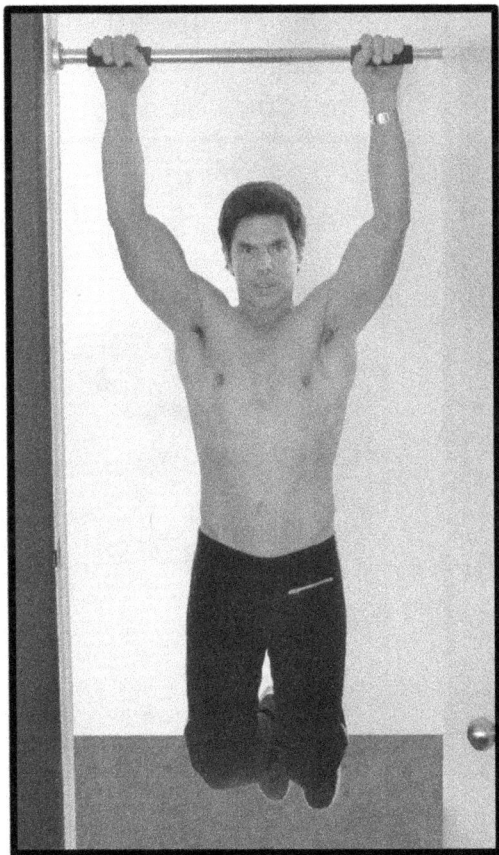

NOTE: We recommend using a chin-up bar that can be installed between a door jam in a room you go through often. Just in case you need reminding to use it.*

*WARNING: Install your chin-up bar **securely.** Cutting a notch in the trim as above is a good idea.*

a) <u>Standard Pull-Ups</u>

(main muscles: biceps, lats, forearms and abs)

With your hands facing toward you, at shoulder width, pull your body up, raising your chin above the bar. Lower back down about half way* and repeat as many times as you are able. Don't be upset if you find this exercise difficult to do, because it is. Just do some whenever you think of it, if you can.

*NOTE: Unless you are doing pull-ups regularly, we don't recommend lowering all the way down.

Hint #1: To make things a little easier, stand on a step stool, a chair or something else that won't move. You can then push up with your feet as needed.

Hint #2: If you put the bar in a doorway that you walk through a lot, you might think of doing pull-ups a lot.

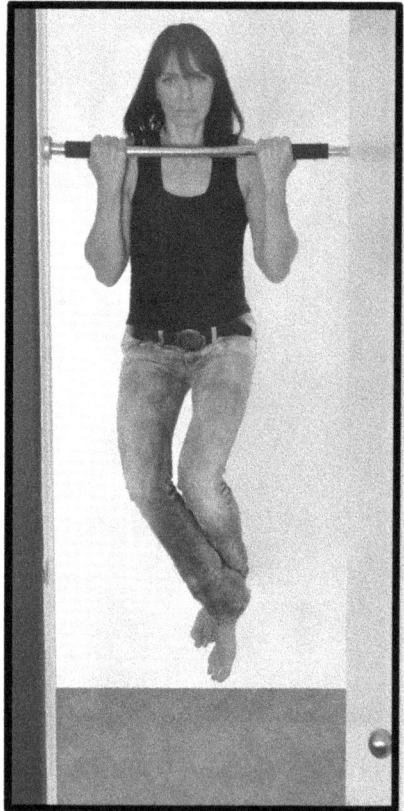

b) <u>Standard Chin-Ups</u>

(main muscles: triceps, lats, forearms and abs)

Grip a chin-up bar with your hands at shoulder width – palms facing away – and pull up with your chin above the bar, just like a pull-up. Again, lower all the way down or as far as you're able and still get back up to repeat. Halfway is enough and it's probably best.

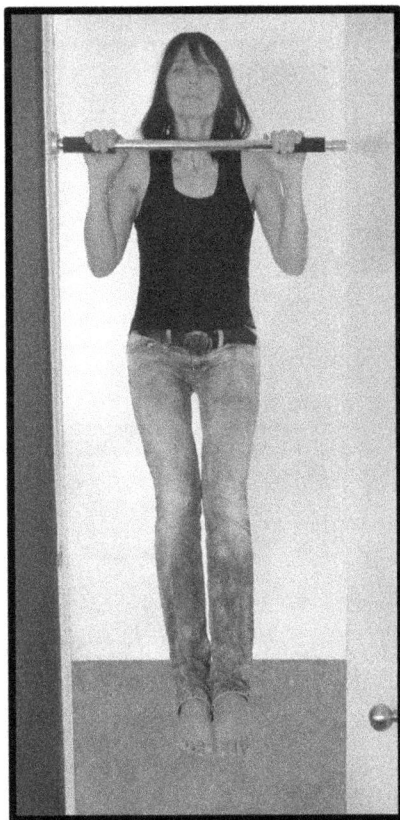

The main difference between chin-ups and pull-ups is that chin-ups utilize your triceps instead of your biceps and... they're harder to do, so whatever you can do is plenty. And if you're able to do more later, go ahead.

NOTE: There's still no strain on Inara's face. That's just not normal, especially when you're holding your position for a picture. In other words, expect this to be difficult, even if Inara isn't showing it.

c) <u>Chin-Up Bar Leg Lifts</u>

(main muscles: stomach, lats and quads)

Version #1: You will need a set of chin-up bar arm straps, as shown. With your elbows resting in the straps, grab the straps near the bar and in a steady motion, bend your legs at the knees and bring them up toward your chest. Try to do this at least five times, then rest. Do more sets when (and if) you can.

Version #2: Twist your torso to either side as you raise your legs, engaging your obliques. Do both sides evenly as above for five reps and more sets *if* you can.

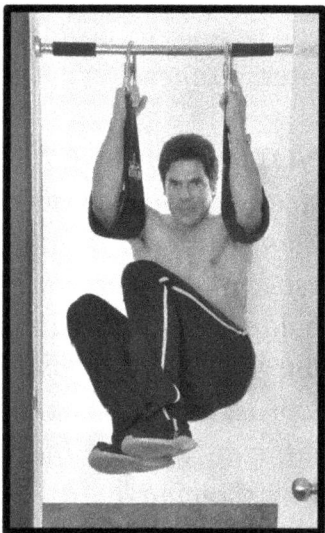

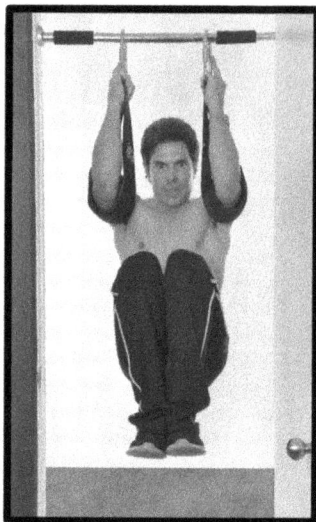

NOTE: *If Billy seems to have a wide-eyed, intense look on his face it's because this move will do that. Try it.*

WARNING: these are very difficult, but very effective.

d) <u>Leg Lift Pull-Ups</u>

(main muscles: stomach, biceps and lats)

These are basically Standard Pull-Ups with added leg lifts: lifting to the front targets your upper abs; lifting and twisting to the sides targets your obliques. Try doing both ways.

Version #1: While doing a pull-up, draw your knees to your chest, lower and repeat.

Version #2: Keeping your knees drawn up to your chest, do as many pull-ups as you can.

Version #3: Keeping your chin above the bar, draw your knees to your chest, lower and repeat.

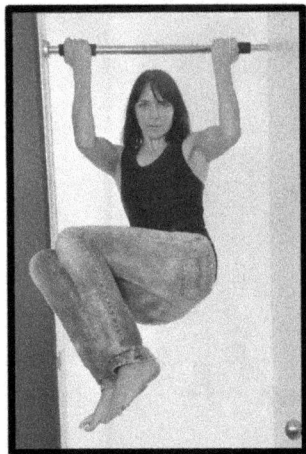

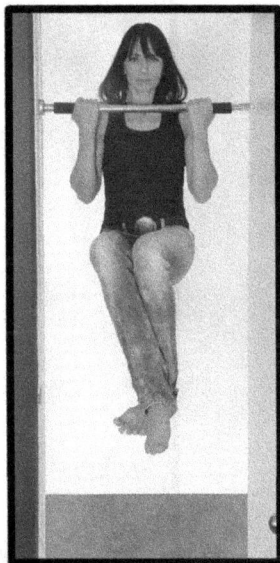

Version #4: With your arms locked at 45 degree angles, draw your knees up to your chest and repeat.

WARNING: They aren't easy.

#6 FULL BODY

All of the exercises in this section are excellent for giving you what's come to be known as "the afterburn effect". In other words, your body continues to burn fat well after you've finished doing the exercise – even while you are asleep. But you do have to do more than just stand there and pose, like Billy and Inara.

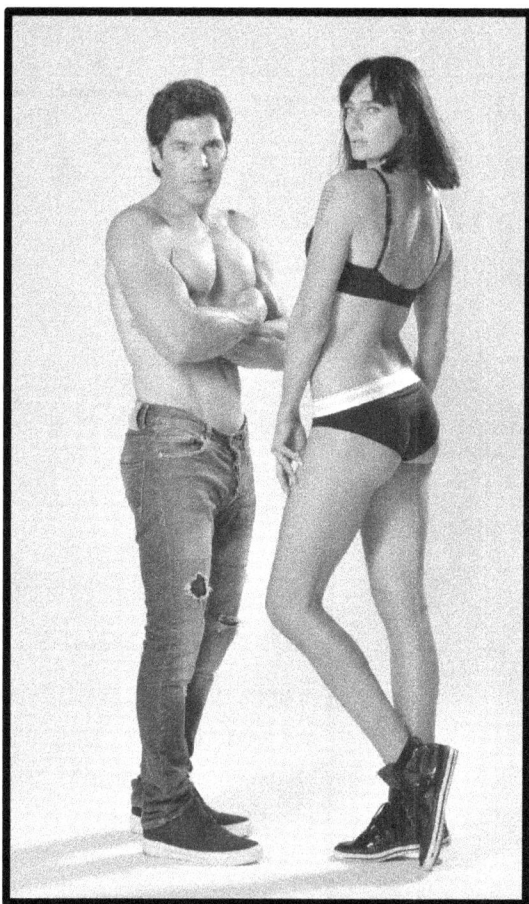

a) <u>Weight Swing</u>

(main muscles: lower back, glutes, quads and shoulders)

Start with a kettle-bell held low with both arms* and your feet apart in a crouched squat position.

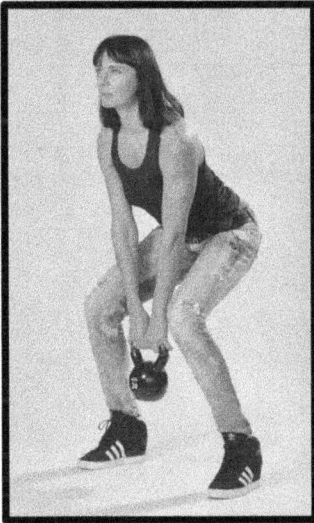

Simultaneously push up with your legs as you swing the weight up to about eye level... and pause.

*can also do one arm at a time.

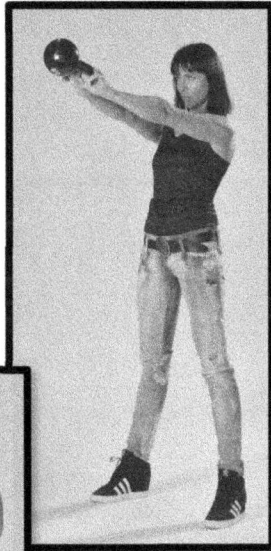

Swing down to the starting position and repeat. Try doing this for ten reps. Take a break before trying another set for a total of three sets.

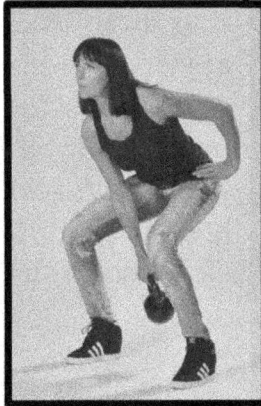

NOTE: *A kettle-bell works best, but a dumbbell or even a sack of potatoes will do.*

b) <u>Burpees</u>

(main muscles: triceps, chest, abs, quads, glutes and calves)

Starting from an upright Push-Up position...

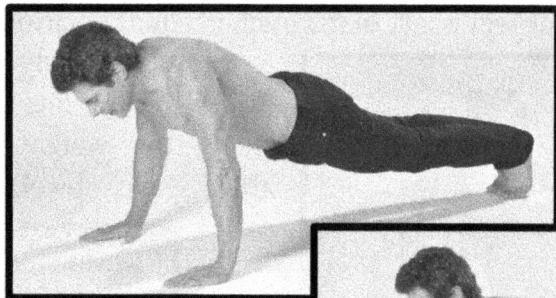

...spring into a crouch on all fours...

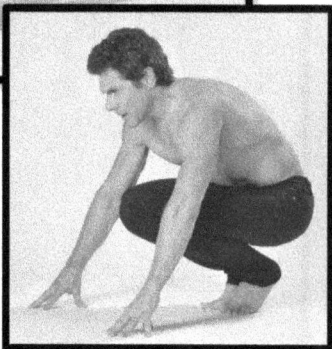

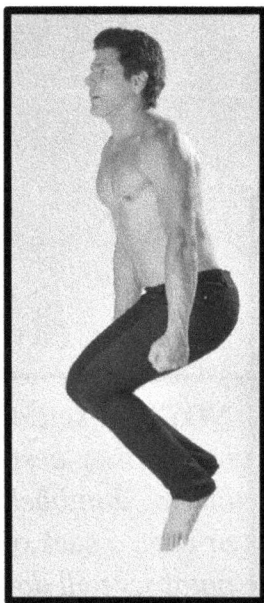

...then hop up quickly and try to bring your knees as close to your chest as you can (which won't be far).

Return to the Push-Up position for five to ten reps. If you're on the floor panting, take a break. Try for three sets. It's not easy, but it's effective.

WARNING: *On a full stomach, "throw-upees" are quite possible.*

c) <u>Mountain Climb</u>

(main muscles: stomach, thighs and various stretches)

Place your hands in a Push-Up position, with one foot forward (knee close to your chest) and the other foot extended straight back.

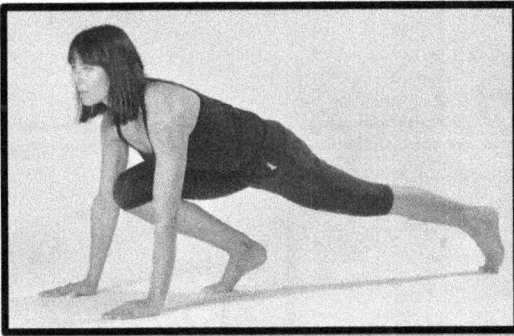

WARNING:
Again, we don't advise doing this on a full stomach.

Keeping your hands in place, quickly alternate your feet in almost a running-in-place motion, for a total of twenty times (ten with each leg). Once you've caught your breath, do two more sets. But be forewarned, <u>this is a very demanding excersise</u>.

NOTE: as you switch your feet your body will arch in more of a "V" shape.

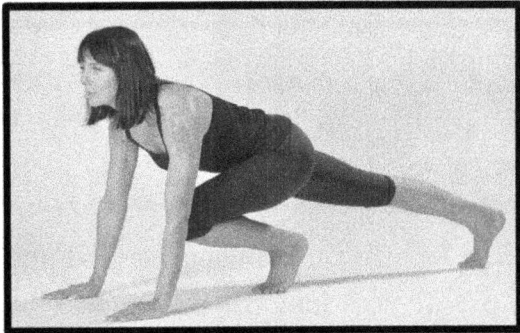

d) <u>Lift, Roll, Push and Jump</u>

(main muscles: abs, glutes, quads, chest, shoulders and lower body)

Part I – Start by lying on your back, with your hands at your hips. Lift your legs straight back over your head to the floor.

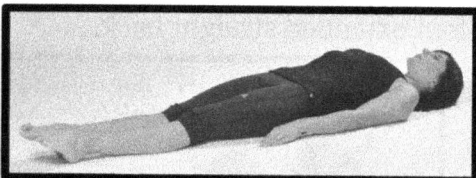

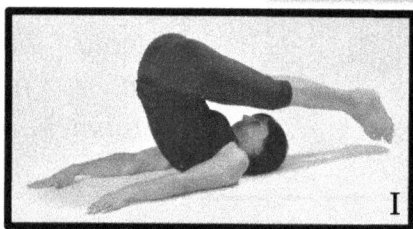

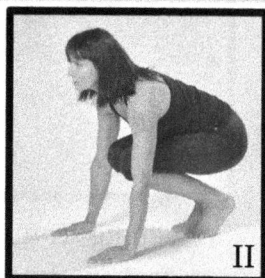

Part II – Roll forward and pop up on all fours.

Part III – Stretch your legs back into a push-up position and push up.

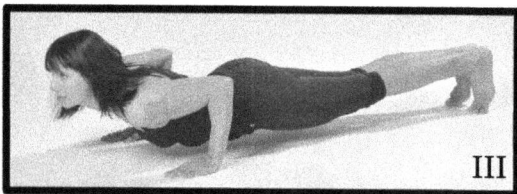

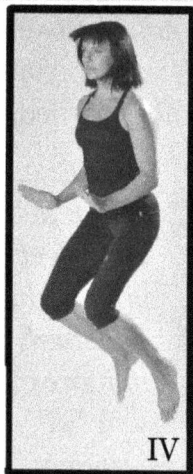

Part IV – Spring to your feet and jump up, with your knees as high as possible.

NOTE: *Repeat if you can, <u>but no more than ten reps</u>.*

#7 AEROBICS

LEVEL III aerobics require more strenuous movement than LEVEL II to increase respiration and heart rate. Such exercises could involve jumping, running, biking, sports and yes, even... sex*.

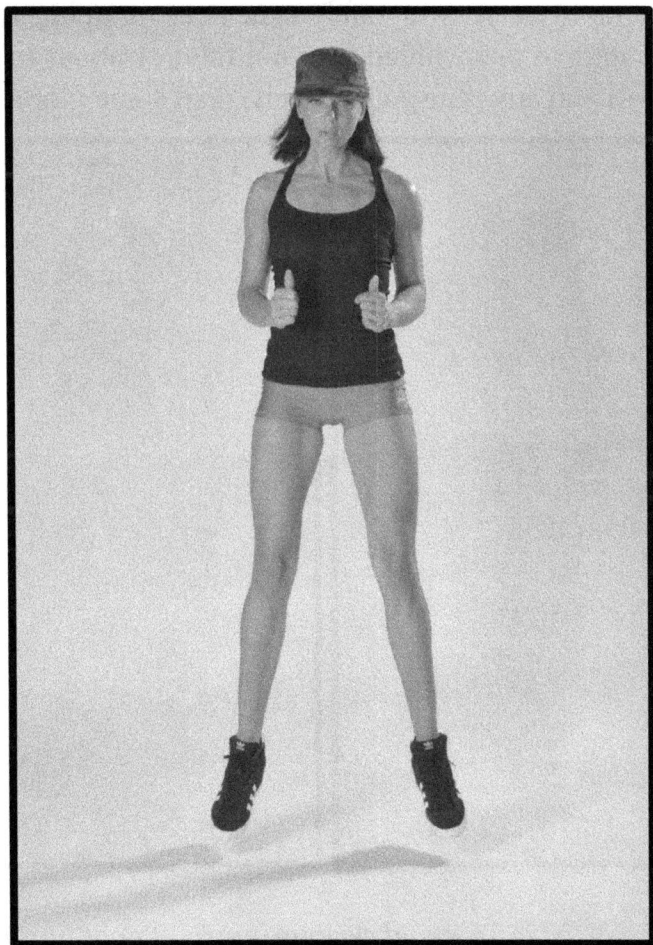

For that, you'll have to use your own imagination.

a) <u>Precision Jumping</u>

(main muscles: lower body)

Place a strip of masking tape on the floor and with both feet together, jump from side to side over the tape, as wide as you safely can. Keep jumping until you start to feel winded (but not faint or about to fall down) and any time you're ready, do it some more.

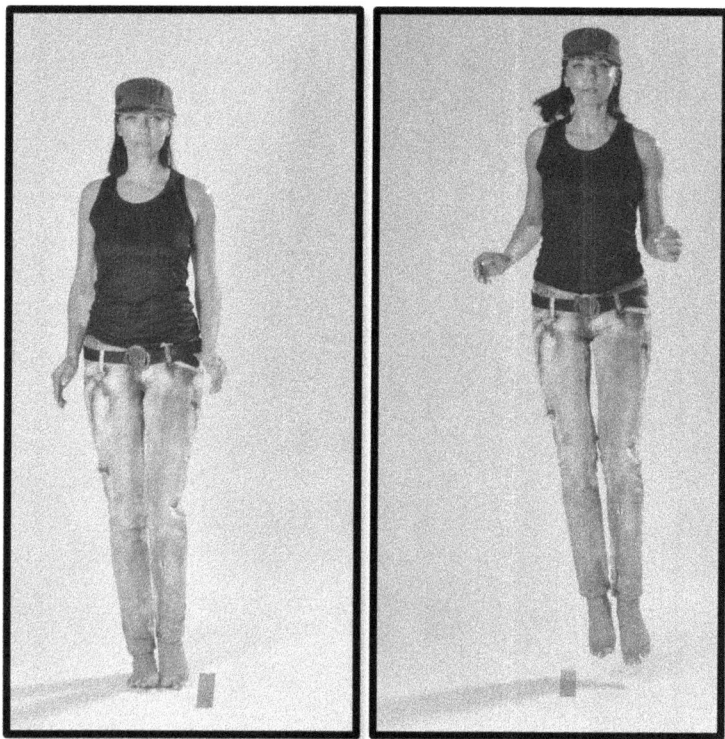

WARNING: *To avoid serious injury, do not jump on any surface or over any object that can move.*

b) <u>Precision Hopping</u>

(main muscles: glutes, quads and calves)

Place masking tape on the floor in the shape of a large plus sign. Hop on both feet* from corner to corner or random patterns. Hop until you almost drop. And do it some more whenever you feel able.

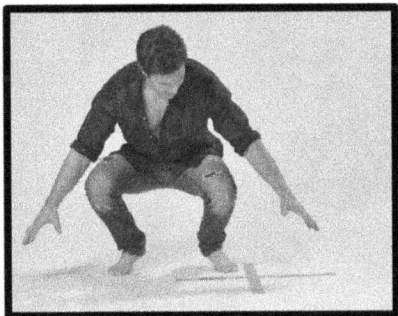

Hint #1: The more you bend down to almost a squat, the more you will engage your quads and butt.

WARNING: Be sure you are hopping over or on a surface that can't move.

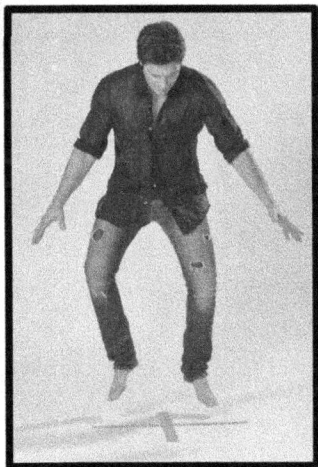

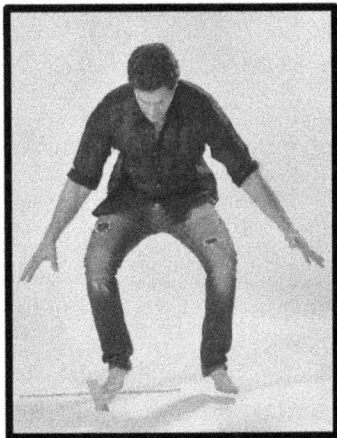

*Hint #2: For extra work on balance, try hopping on one leg at a time. But <u>this is extra hard to do.</u>

c) <u>Jumping Rope</u>

(main muscles: glutes, thighs and calfs)

Using a jump rope... jump rope.

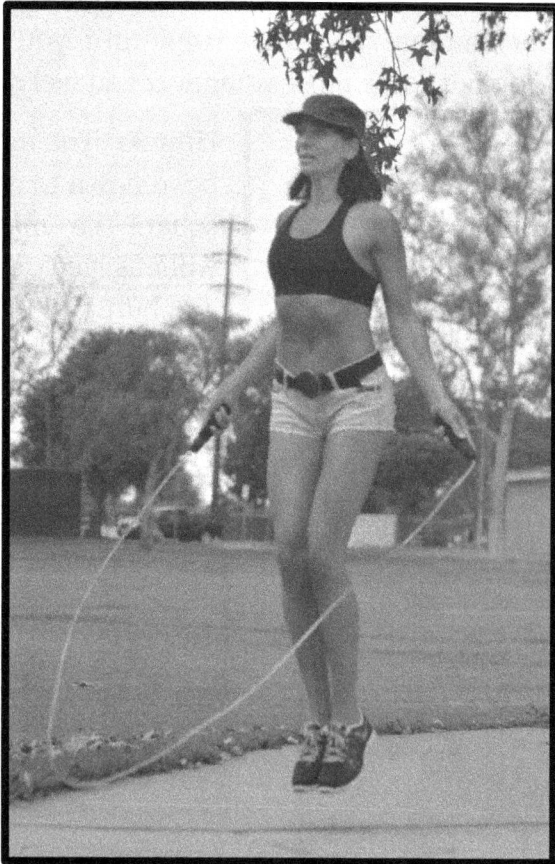

This exercise involves getting into a rhythm, so do what works for you. And do it as long as you feel comfortable. It can be quite a workout.

d) <u>Running in Place</u>*

(main muscles: butt, thighs, stomach)

If you're doing it right, this exercise is quite tiring. It is however, just what it says. Without any forward movement, raise your knees up as high as you can and "run" as fast as you can for about ten steps. Maybe mix in some Jumping Jacks between sets. And do as many sets as you can without overdoing it.

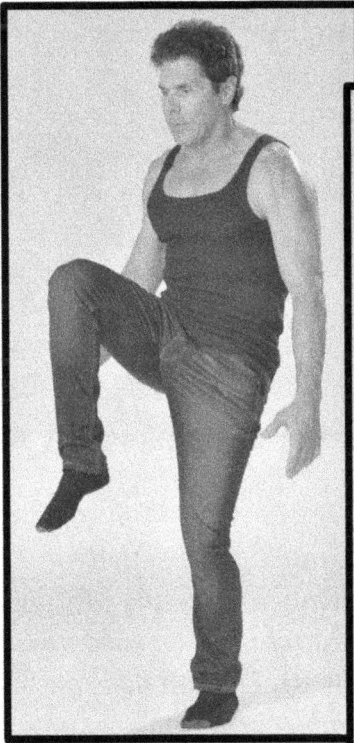

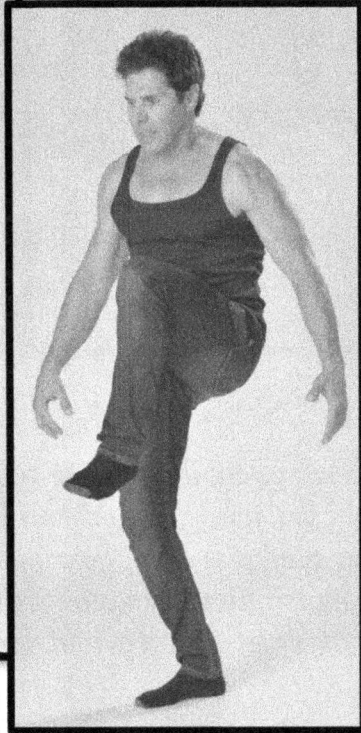

NOTE: *Billy is lifting his knees extremely high in these two pictures...*   *all pictures taken 2017

...and from the looks of him in the two pictures below, he <u>might be</u> extremely high.

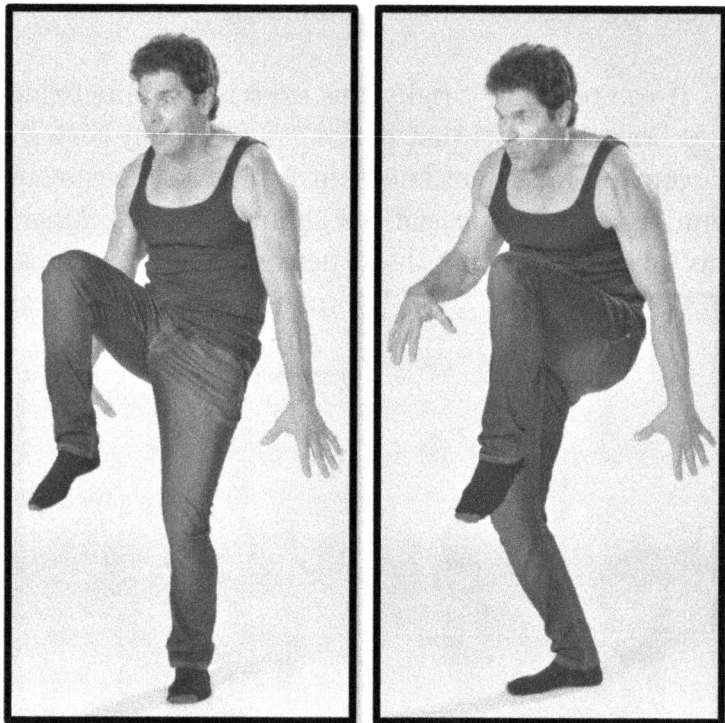

<u>CAUTION:</u> *Running in place can be a high exertion exercise, so if you are feeling light headed or too winded, take a break. And if you are feeling just plain too silly, like Billy, you might want to be sure no one is watching (or taking pictures). Though he is getting some pretty good height on his lifts.*

e) <u>Running (fast) – Cycling (distance) – Sports (challenge)</u>

(main muscles: whole body)

These activities should need no clarifying, except to say that in LEVEL III, they aren't meant to be done leisurely. While any attempt may be better than nothing, that's not the goal here. So, if you really want the most out of them, then try to give them your all.

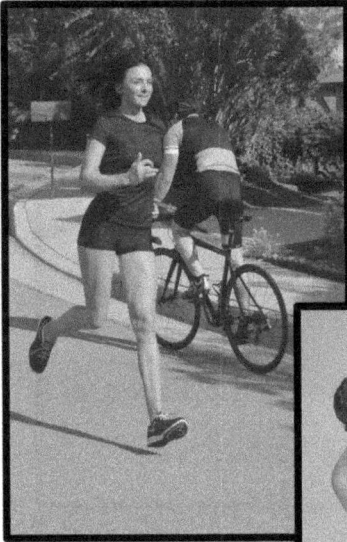

Hint: if you have trouble finding the motivation for any of these activities, a partner* might help.

*Rule #1: You (Billy) should always choose – or pick on -- someone your own size.

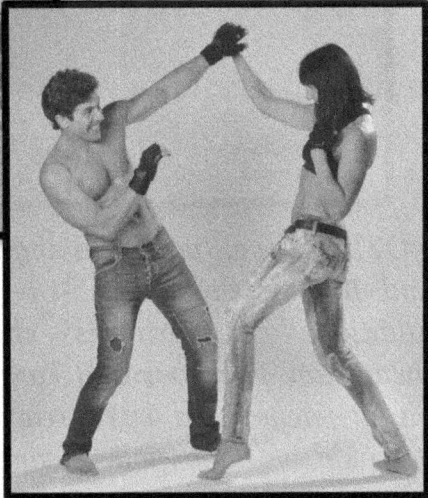

#8 DUO EXERCISES

There are always exercises that can be done simultaneously, like some of those listed in the previous group of Aerobics, but the ones included here utilize the help of a partner – except of course for the one below which is not a fair depiction because again, Inara is doing all the balancing.

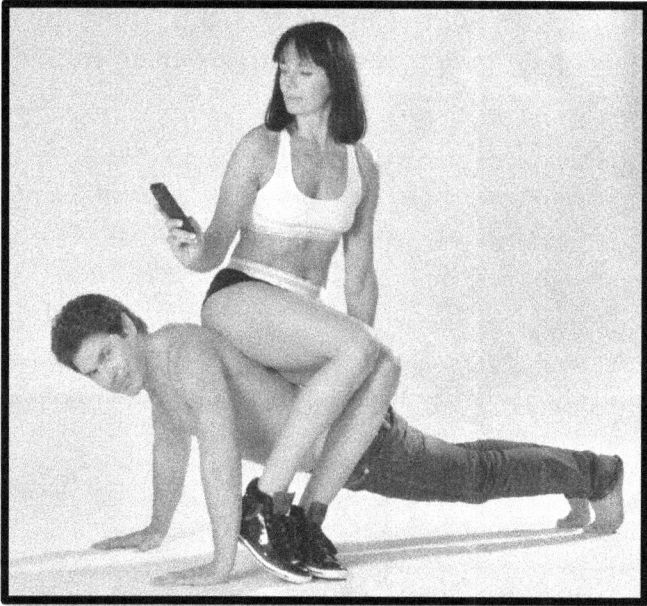

NOTE: *Above, Inara is doing Squats with an assist and Billy is doing Push-Ups with added weight. Additionally, Inara is checking her Email, Instagram, Facebook and Twitter. This one is also a bit far-fetched and isn't a true Duo Exercise because it would be impossible to switch positions. Billy is lousy with the Internet.*

a) <u>Duo Neck Lifts</u>

(main muscles: neck)

While on a mat and propped up on your elbows, tip your head all the way back. With a partner's hand resisting on your forehead, bring your neck forward until it's straight up. Now do the same move with your neck turned to the sides.

Perform these at your own pace for about ten reps each. No need to do more.

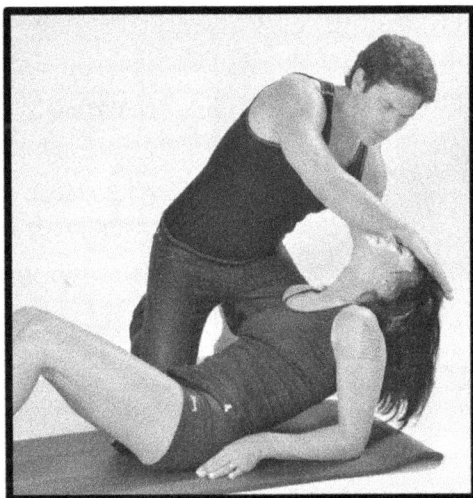

Partners allow for an even more thorough workout than a Medicine-Ball Neck Lift, with the addition of resistance over the full range of the move.

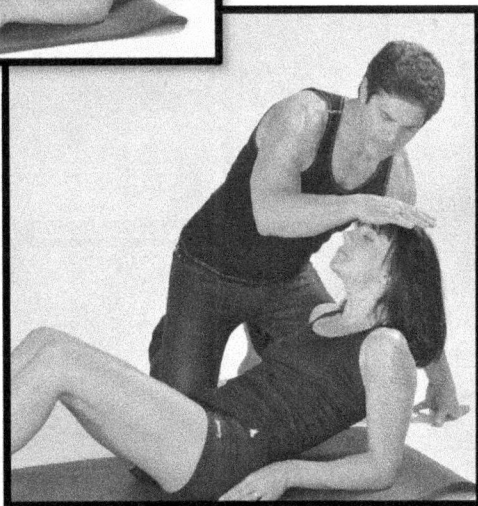

b) <u>Duo Upper Leg Lifts</u>

(main muscles: thighs and abs)

    While lying down, clench your quads and abs hard as you slowly raise your legs for a good moving clench and your partner resists along the way, *at your own pace.* Increase or decrease the resistance or try raising one leg at a time to alter the workout.

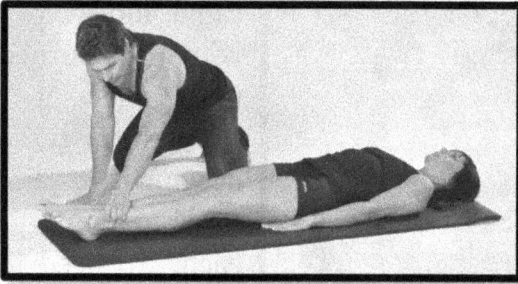

See also: LEVEL I, #12 DUO CLENCHES – e) Duo Upper Leg/Abs Clenches.

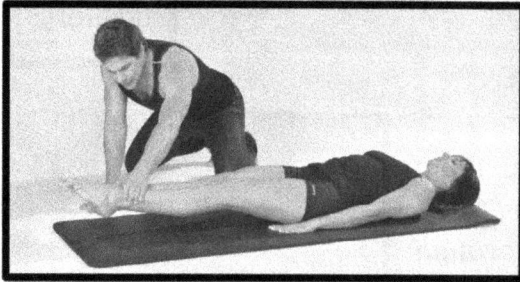

When you have done as many as you can, switch positions with your partner.

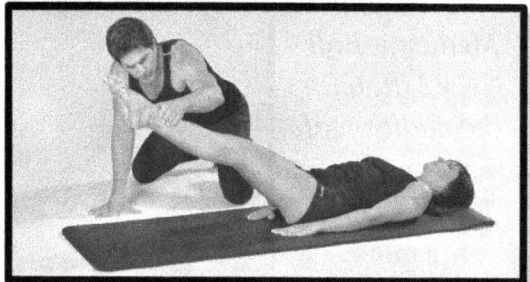

c) <u>Duo See-Saw</u>

(main muscles: hamstrings, abs, and back)

While sitting on a mat facing each other, at arms' length, grip hands with your partner. Keeping your arms straight, one of you pulls back while the other provides resistance as they are pulled forward.

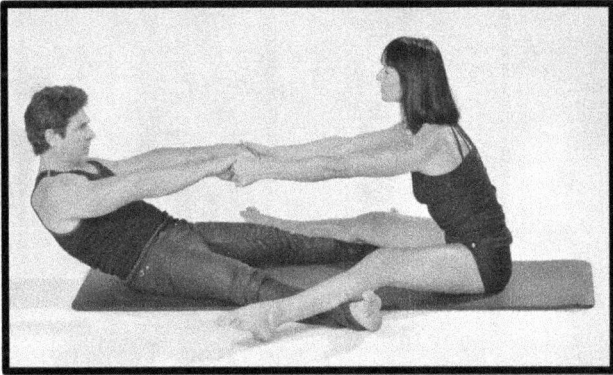

Pulling back mainly uses your abs and hamstrings while resisting mainly uses your abs and back. Now reverse the process, until one of you has had enough.

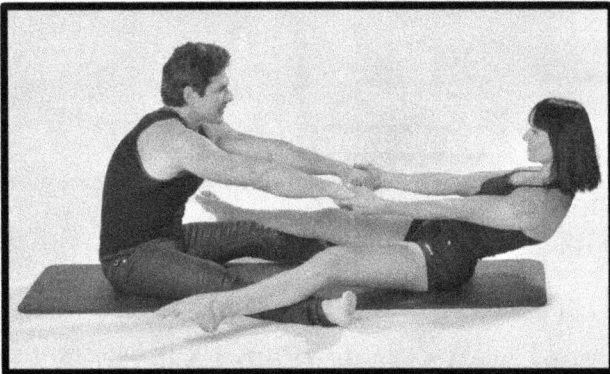

Daily/Weekly Exercise Suggestions (LEVEL III)

By LEVEL III you should be doing several **Xer-tasks** daily using your butt and stomach muscles at least, but hopefully more. And if you haven't yet started doing some workout routines, think about it.

<u>Lunges</u>

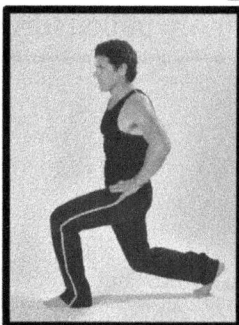
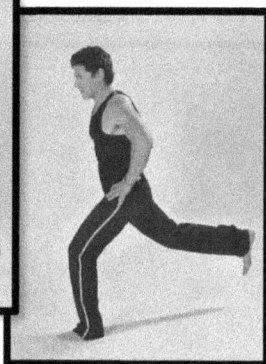

Lunge Walking
(Version #1)
(S1-L III-1c)

Lunge Walking
(Version #2) (S1-L III-1c)

<u>Crunches and Various Ab Exercises</u>

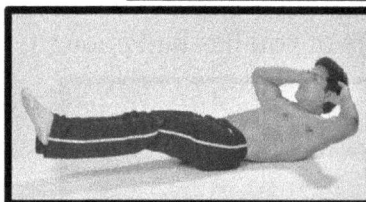
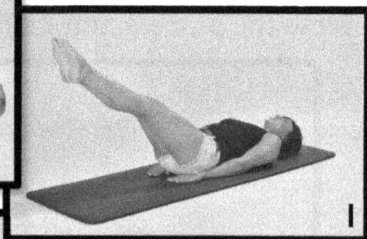

Elevated
Crunch
(S1-L III-2a)

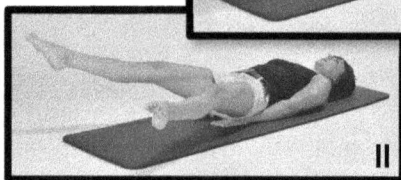

Scissor Leg Lifts Combo (Parts I & II) (S1-L III-2e)

Biceps, Triceps, Shoulders and Lats

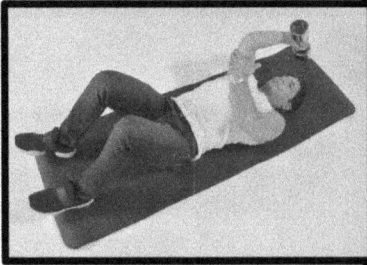

Triceps Press (w/weight)
(with support) (S1-L III-4j)

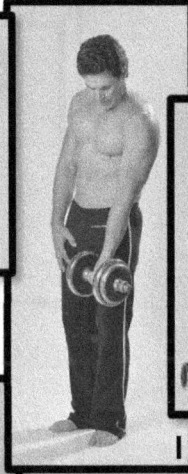

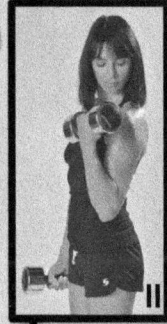

Curls (Parts I & II)
(S1-L III-4a)

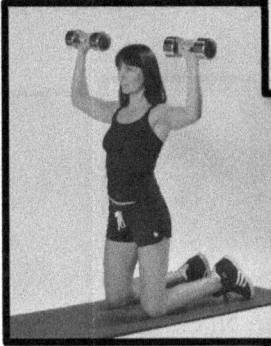

Shoulder Press
(S1-L III-4d)

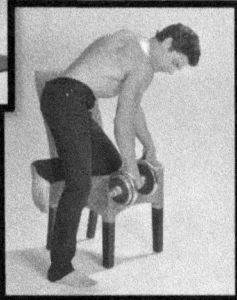

Push-Ups

Lats Pull (S1-L III-4g)

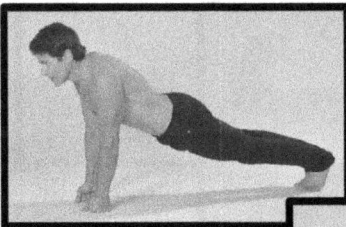

Advanced Push-Ups
(Version #1)
(S1-L III-3a)

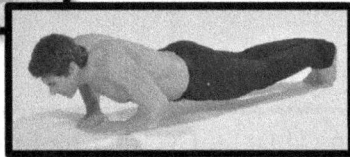

Advanced Push-Ups (Version #2) (S1-L III-3a)

Pull-Ups

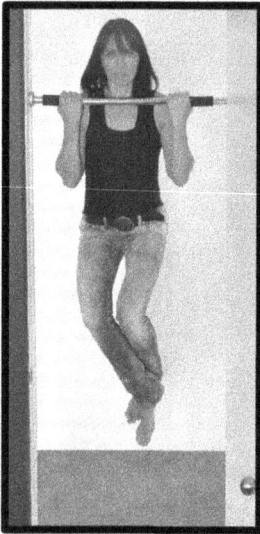

Full Body

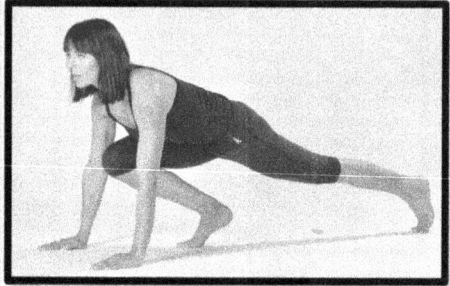

Mountain Climb
(S1-L III-6c)

Duo Exercises

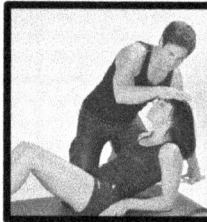

Standard
Pull-Ups
(S1-L III-5a)

Duo Neck Lifts
(S1-L III-8a)

Aerobics

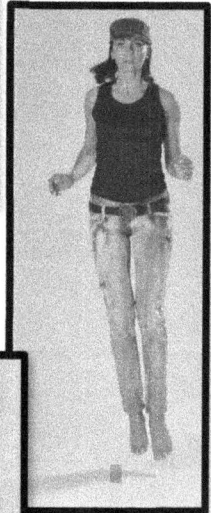

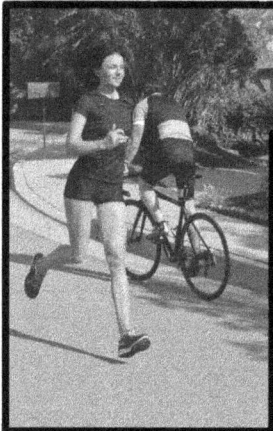

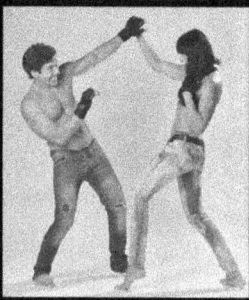

Precision
Jumping
(S1-L III-7a)

Running (fast) – Cycling (distance) –
Sports (challenge) (S1-L III-7e)

STAGE 2
(Beginner Exercise Routines)

For those of you ready for **Xer-task** routines using the exercises from STAGE 1, LEVEL I, the following routines offer examples of some suggested workouts. You can also make substitutions or choose workouts of your own, just make sure that you have a specific plan for either targeting a particular muscle group or performing more of a mixed muscle workout. And remember, unless you're working a large muscle like the butt or stomach or you're doing aerobics or whole body moves, then vary the muscle groups used. Muscles require time to rebuild, especially the smaller ones. So, if you do biceps one day don't do them the day after. Regardless, if you don't choose Billy and Inara's picks, you can still utilize them as a guide. Now, get going.

NOTE: *The individual exercises in the Stage 2 Routines (and also in the Stage 3 and Stage 4 Routines) are numerically labeled mainly for the purposes of identification and are not necessarily intended as the order in which they should be performed. Feel free to do them however you prefer.*
Each exercise is also labeled for easy reference.
Example:
Standing-Still Butt Clench (S1-L I-1a) refers to:
    STAGE 1, LEVEL I, exercise 1a

Workout #1A

<u>The Butt</u>

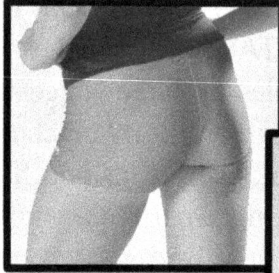

1

Standing-Still
Butt Clench
(S1-L I-1a)

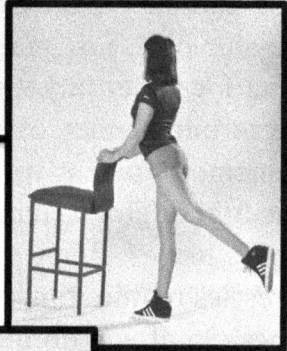

2

Standing
Butt Clench
Leg Lifts
(Balancing)
(S1-L I-1d)

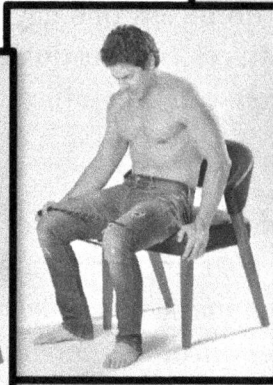

3

Sitting
Hip Abductor
Clench
(S1-L I-1g)

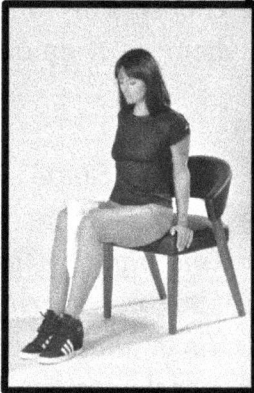

4

Sitting Hip
Adductor Clench
(S1-L I-9d)

Xer-tasking

Workout #1B

The Butt

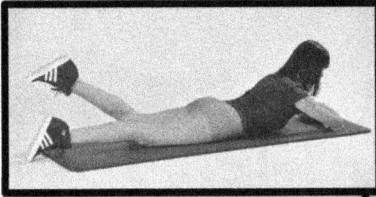

1

Lying-Down
Leg-Lift Clench
(S1-L I-1f)

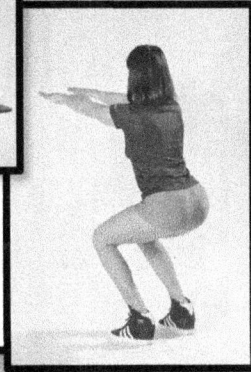

2

Butt Clench
Squats
(S1-L I-1c)

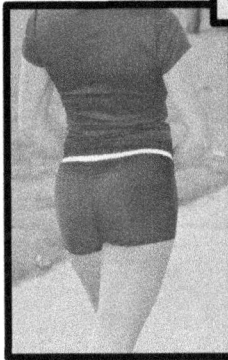

3

Walking
Butt Clench
(S1-L I-1b)

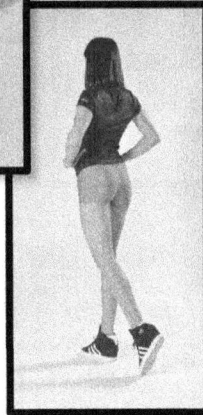

4

Standing Butt Clench
Leg Lifts (Freestanding)
(S1-L I-1d)

Workout #2

The Stomach

1

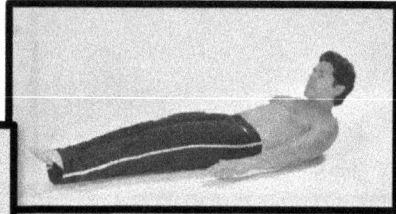

Stomach Clench Crunch
(Lying Down)
(S1-L I-2a)

2

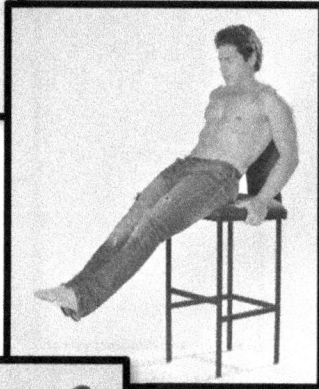

Stomach
Clench
(Standing)
(S1-L I-2a)

3

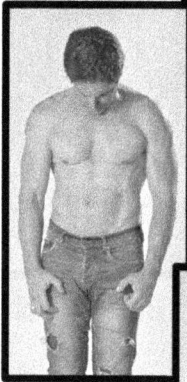

Stomach
Clench
(Sitting)
(S1-L I-2a)

4

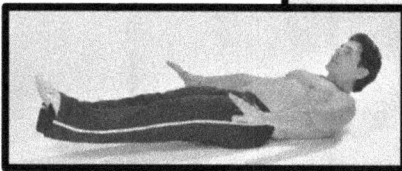

Stomach Clench Crunch
(Lying Down) (with a Leg Lift)
(S1-L I-2a)

Workout #3A

Butt and Stomach

1

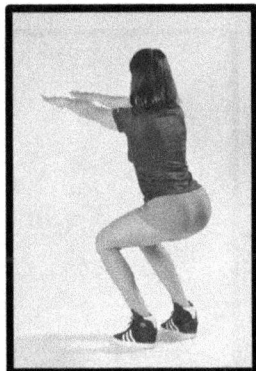

Butt Clench
Squats
(S1-L I-1c)

2

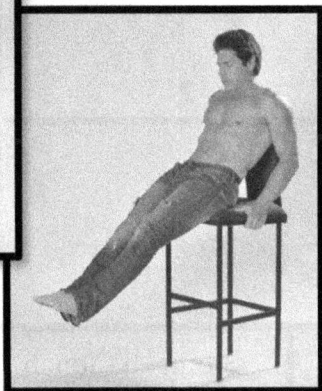

Stomach
Clench
(Sitting)
(S1-L I-2a)

3

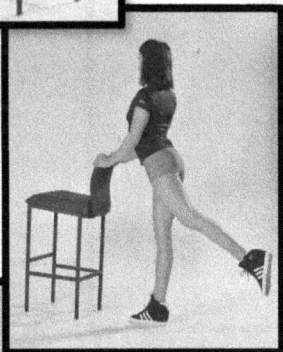

4

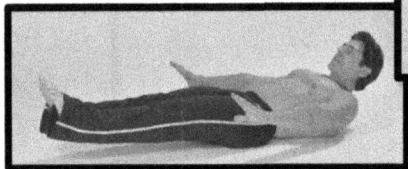

Stomach Clench Crunch
(Lying Down) (with a Leg Lift)
(S1-L I-2a)

Standing
Butt Clench
Leg Lifts
(Balancing)
(S1-L I-1d)

Workout #3B

Butt and Stomach

1

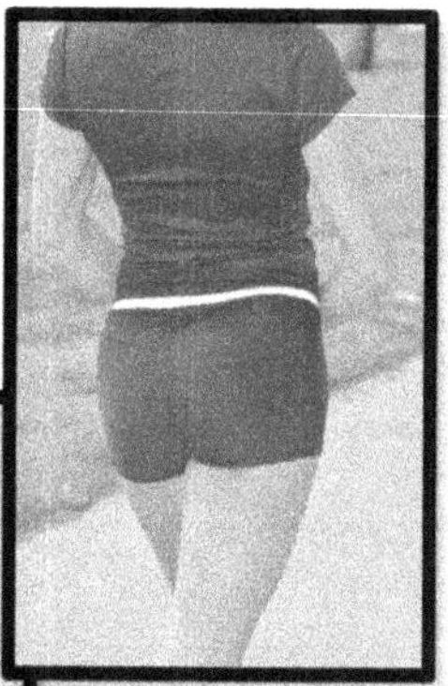

Walking
Butt Clench
(S1-L I-1b)

2

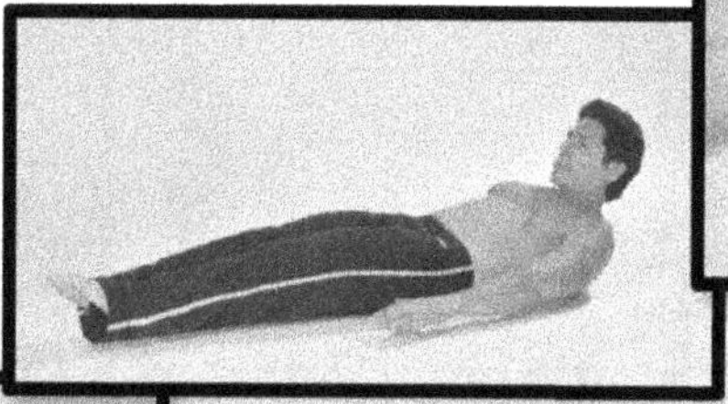

Stomach Clench
Crunch
(Lying Down)
(S1-L I-2a)

3

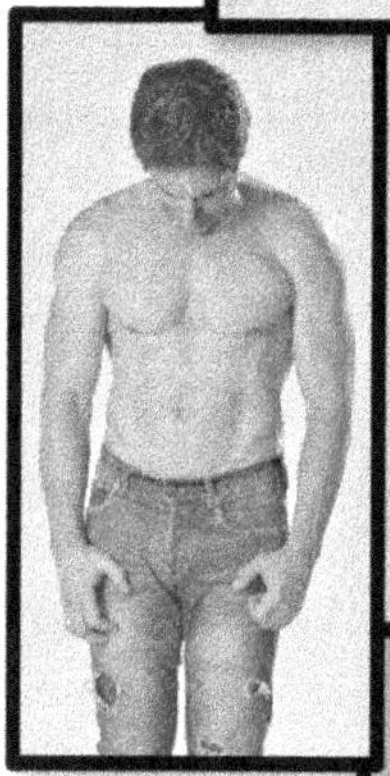

Stomach
Clench
(Standing)
(S1-L I-2a)

4

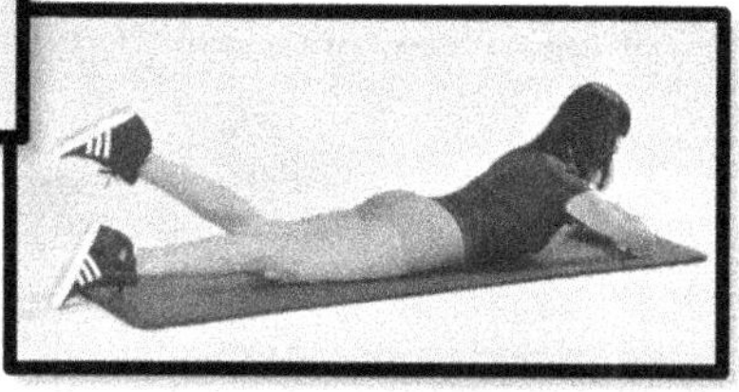

Lying-Down
Leg-Lift Butt Clench
(S1-L I-1f)

Workout #4

Upper Body

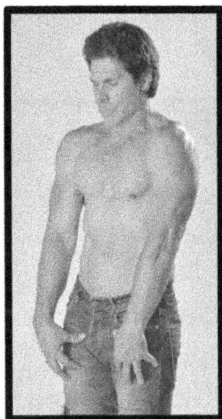

1 Stationary Chest Clench (Version #1) (S1-L I-4a)

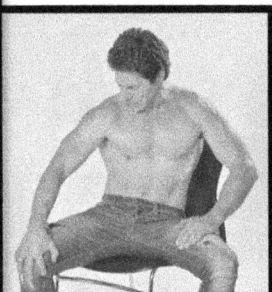

2 Stationary Lats Clench (sitting) (S1-L I-5a)

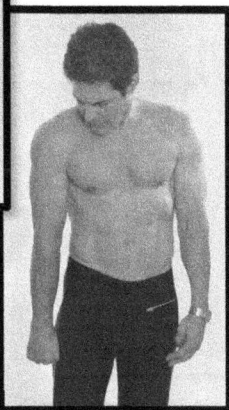

3 Side Forearm Clench S1-L I-8b)

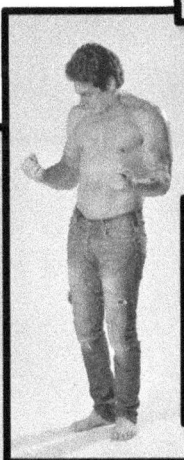

4 Curl Clench Pump (S1-L I-3a)

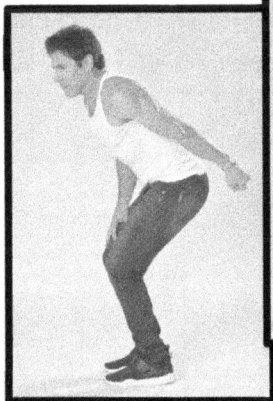

5 Stationary Triceps Clench (S1-L I-7a)

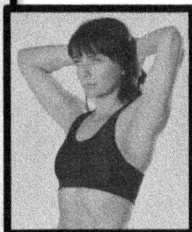

6 Neck Push Clench S1-L I-6a)

Workout #5A

<u>Lower Body</u>

1

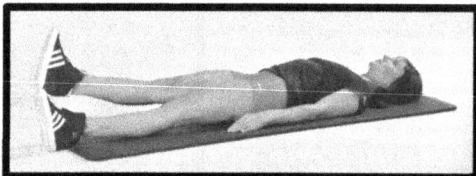

Lying Down Upper-Leg
Clench (Version #2) (S1-L I-9b)

2

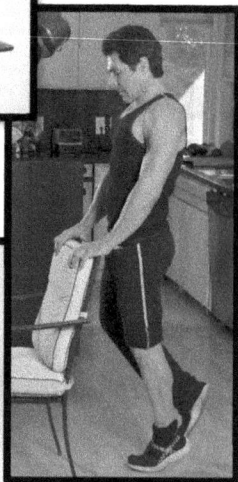

3

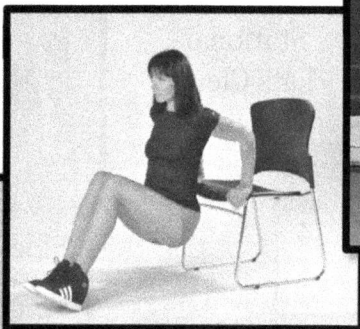

4

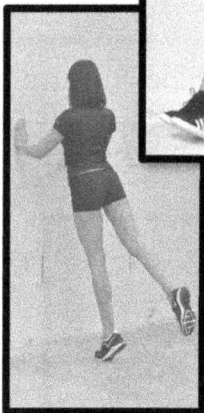

Rising
Calf Clench
(S1-L I-10a)

Chair Butt Clench
(Version #2)
(S1-L I-1e)

Standing
Butt Clench
Leg Lifts
(leaning)
(S1-L I-1d)

Workout #5B

Lower Body

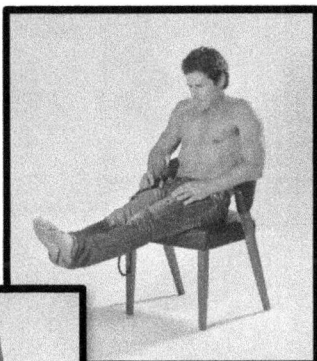

Sitting Upper-Leg Clench (Version #1) (S1-L I-9a)

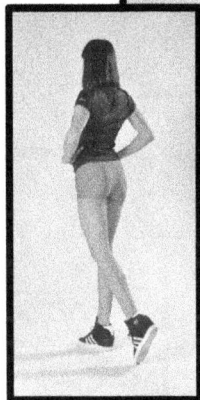

Standing Butt Clench Leg Lifts (Freestanding) (S1-L I-1d)

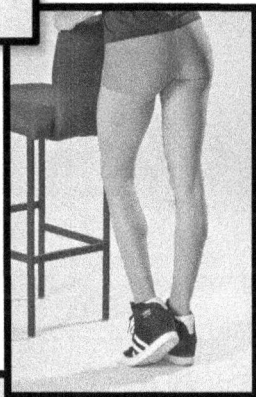

Rising Calf Clench (S1-L I-10a)

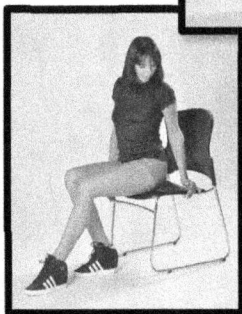

Chair Butt Clench (Version #1) (S1-L I-1e)

Workout #6A

Whole Body

2

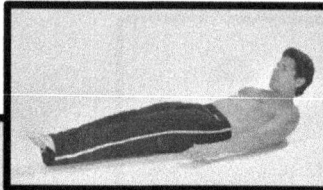

1

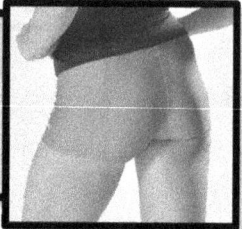

3

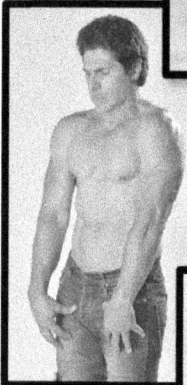

Stomach Clench
Crunch
(Lying Down)
(S1-L I-2a)

Standing-Still
Butt Clench
(S1-L I-1a)

4

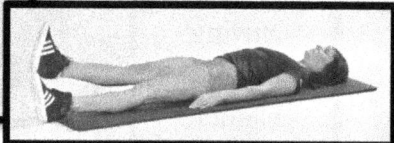

5

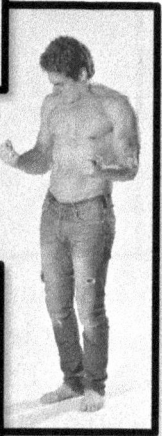

Stationary
Chest
Clench
(Version #1)
(S1-L I-4a)

Lying Down
Upper-Leg Clench
(Version #2) (S1-L I-9b)

6

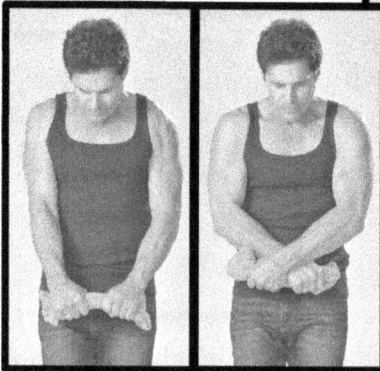

Curl
Clench
Pump
(S1-L I-3a)

Triceps Pull/Push Clench (S1-L I-7b)

Workout #6B

<u>Whole Body</u>

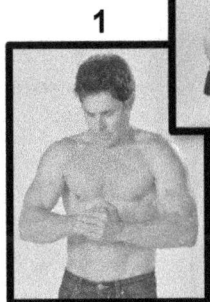

1 Stationary Chest Clench (Version #2) (S1-L I-4a)

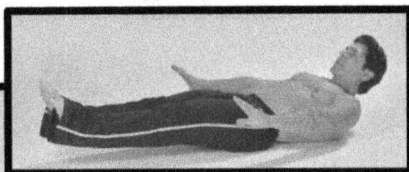

2 Stomach Clench Crunch (Lying Down) (with a leg lift) (S1-L I-2a)

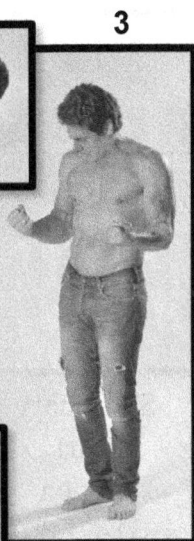

3 Curl Clench Pump (S1-L I-3a)

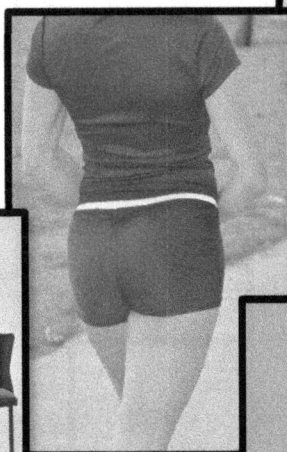

4 Walking Butt Clench (S1-L I-1b)

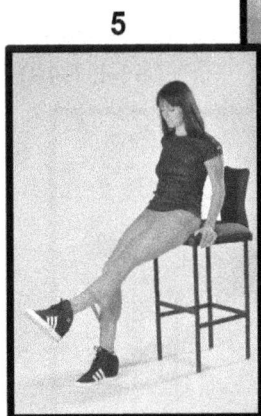

5 Sitting Upper-Leg Clench (Version #2) (S1-L I-9a)

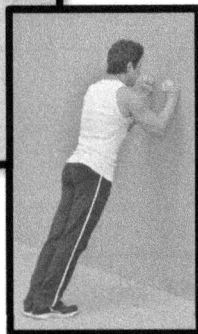

6 Triceps Push-Back Clench (S1-L I-7c)

Workout #6C

Whole Body

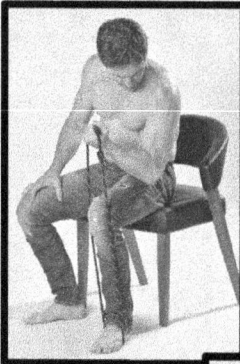

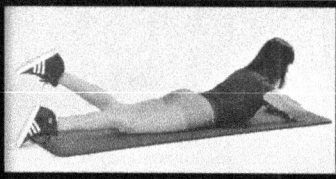

Lying-Down
Leg-Lift Butt Clench
(S1-L I-1f)

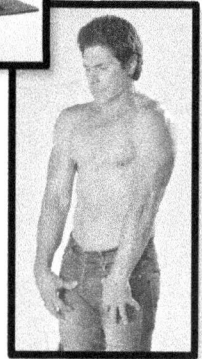

Stationary
Curl
Clench
(S1-L I-3b)

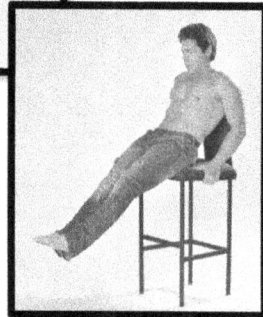

Stationary
Chest Clench
(Version #1)
(S1-L I-4a)

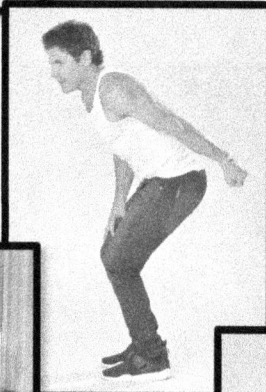

Stationary
Tricep
Clench
(S1-L I-7a)

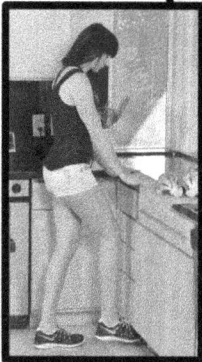

Pushing
Upper-Leg Clench
(Version #1)
(S1-L I-9c)

Stomach Clench
(Sitting)
(S1-L I-2a)

Workout #6D

<u>Whole Body</u>

1

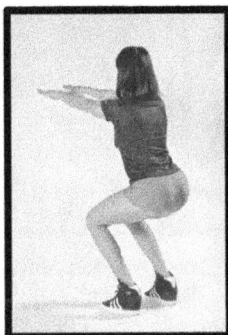

Butt Clench
Squats
(S1-L I-1c)

3

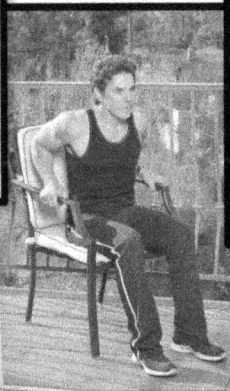

Lats Lift
Clench
(S1-L I-5b)

2

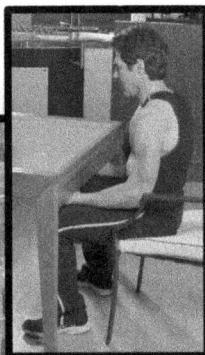

Stationary
Curl Clench
(Version 2)
(S1-L I-3b)

4

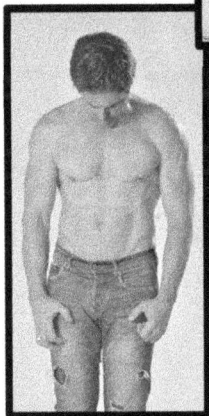

Stomach
Clench
(Standing)
(S1-L I-2a)

5

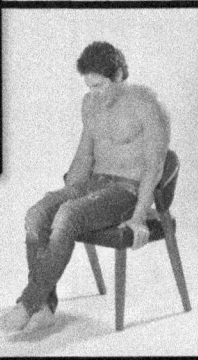

6

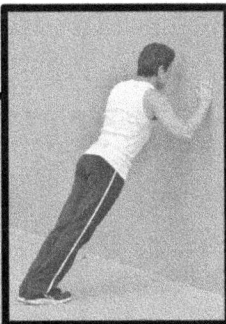

Leaning
Chest Clench
(S1-L I-4b)

Pushing Upper-Leg Clench (Version #2) (S1-L I-9c)

Additions and Substitutions
(Part 1)

Thighs

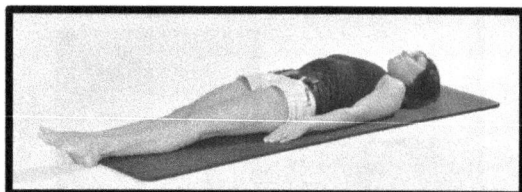

Lying Down Upper-Leg
Clench (Version #1)
(S1-L I-9b)

Lats

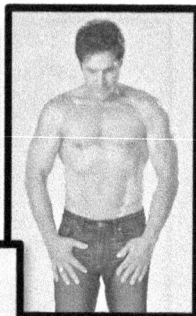

Stationary
Lats Clench
(open hand)
(S1-L I-5a)

Forearms

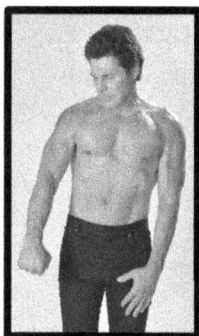

Freestyle
Forearm
Clench
(Version #1)
(S1-L I-8a)

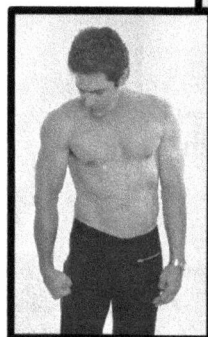

Stationary
Lats Clench
(closed fist)
(S1-L I-5a)

Kegels

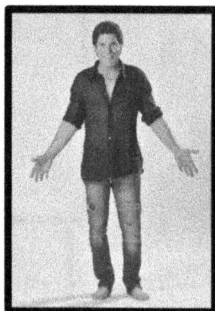

Kegel Clench (S1-L I-11a)*

Chest

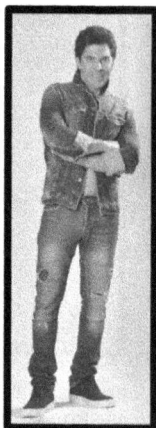

Casual
Chest Clench
(S1-L I-4c)

*Don't overlook muscles you can't see... like Kegels.

Additions and Substitutions
(Part 2)

Duo Exercises

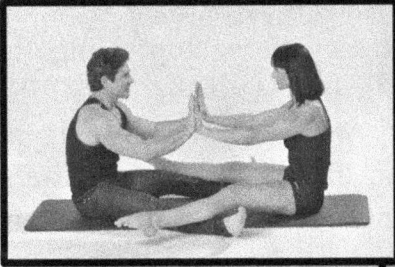

Duo Sitting Abs/Chest
Press Clench (S1-L I-12a)

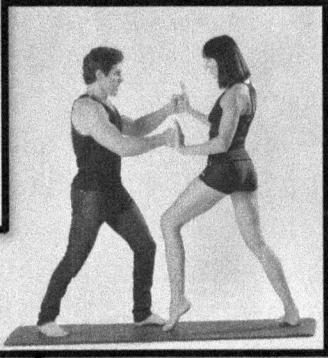

Duo Standing
Abs/Chest/Thighs/
Butt Clench
(S1-L I-12b)

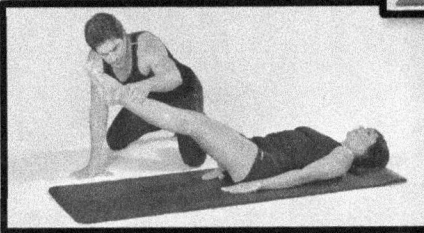

Duo Upper-Leg/Abs
Clench (S1-L I-12e)

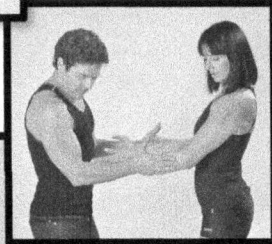

Duo Standing
Chest/Triceps
Press Clench
(S1-L I-12c)

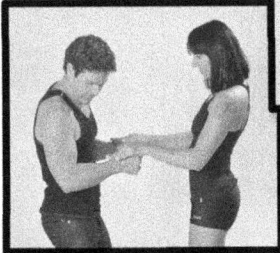

Duo Standing Biceps/Chest
Press Clench (S1-L I-12d)

STAGE 3
(Intermediate Exercise Routines)

Just because you are ready for STAGE 3, LEVEL 2 exercise routines is no reason to stop doing the isometrics of STAGE 1, LEVEL 1 or STAGE 2 whenever you can. They will help keep you in an exercising frame of mind. In fact, think of STAGE 3 and STAGE 4 as additions to, instead of substitutions for, STAGE 2.

Now that your head is spinning, keep up the momentum. And there is no harm in doing more. So, if you can, then do it.

Workout #1A

Butt and Lower Body

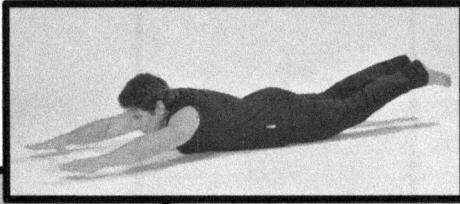

Superman
(S1-L II-1i)

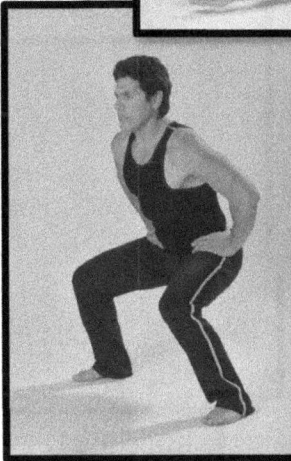

Standard Squats
(S1-L II-1a)

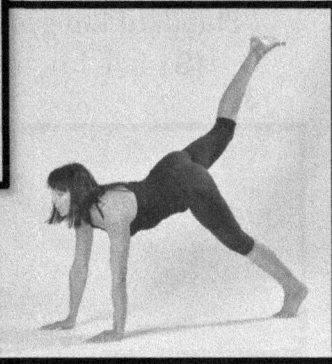

Backward
Leg Lifts
(Version #2)
(S1-L II-1f)

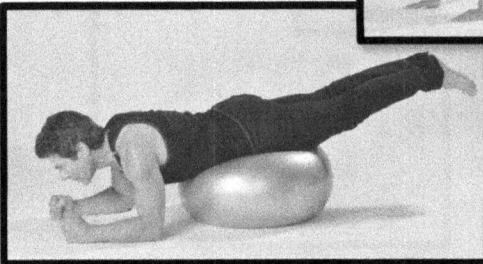

Medicine-Ball Plank (S1-L II-1h)

Workout #1B

1   <u>Butt and Lower Body</u>

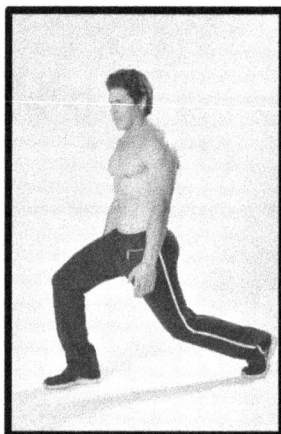

Standard Lunges
(S1-L II-1d)

2

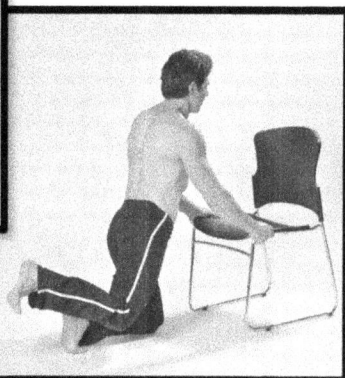

Kneeling Leg-Lifts
(S1-L II-1e)

3

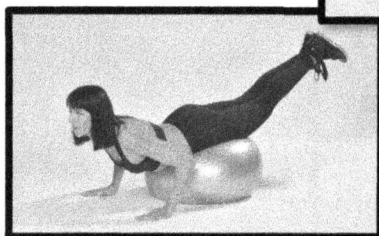

Medicine-Ball
Backward
Leg Lifts
(S1-L II-1g)

4

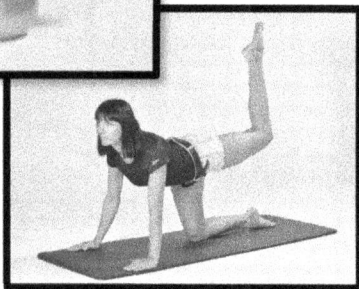

Backward Leg-Lifts (Version #1)
(S1-L II-1f)

Workout #1C

Butt and Lower Body

1

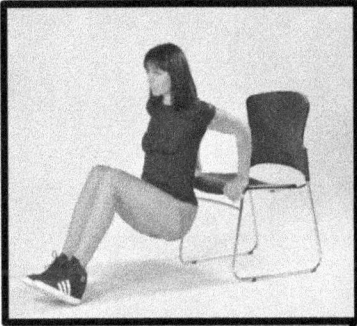

Chair Squats
(S1-L II-1c)

2

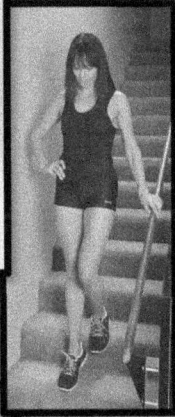

Stairway
Butt Lifts
(S1-L II-1j)

3

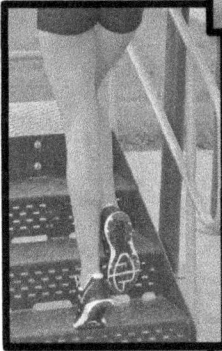

Stairway
Calf Lift
(S1-L II-1k)

4

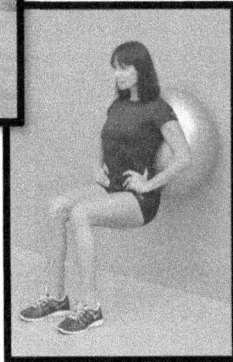

Medicine-Ball Wall Squats
(S1-L II-1b)

Workout #2A

Stomach and Thighs

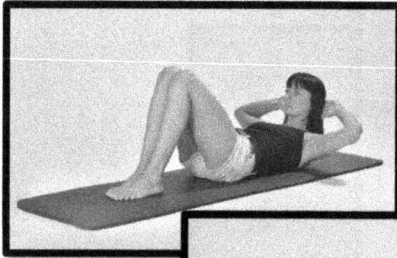

1

Standard
Crunch
(S1-L II-2a)

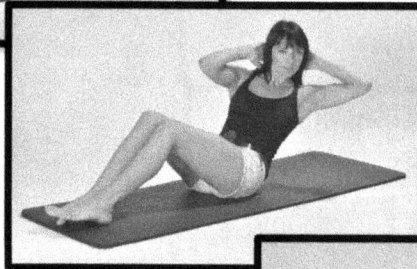

2

Standard
Crunch
(with a twist)
(S1-L II-2b)

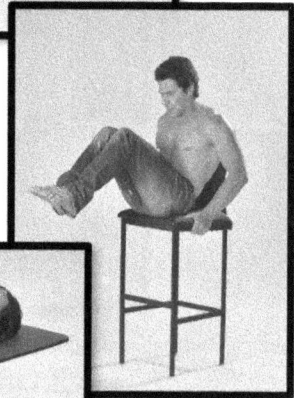

3

Forward
Leg-Lifts
(Sitting)
(Version #1)
(S1-L II-2f)

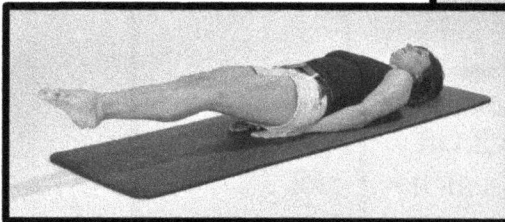

4

Forward Leg-Lifts (Lying Down)
(S1-L II-2e)

Workout #2B

Stomach and Thighs

1

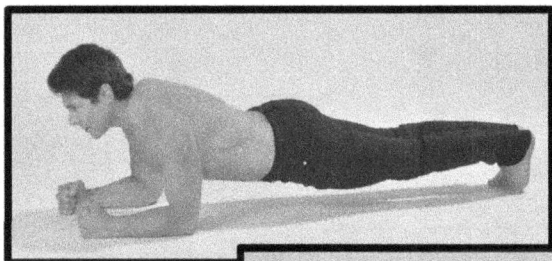

The Plank
(S1-L II-2c)

2

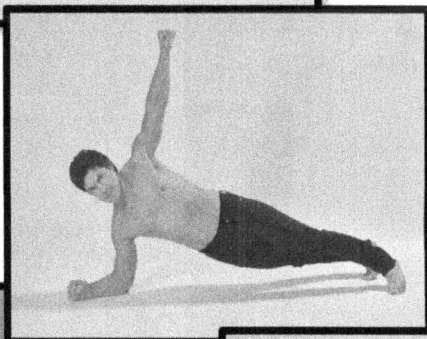

The
Twisting
Plank
(S1-L II-2d)

3

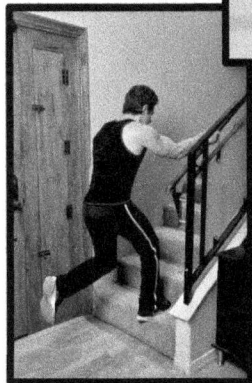

Stairway
Thigh Lifts
(S1-L II-2g)

4

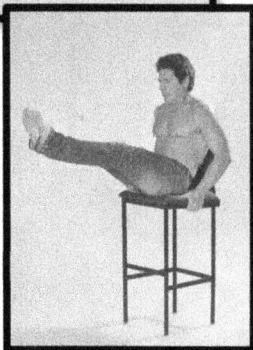

Forward Leg-Lifts
(Sitting) (Version #2)
(S1-L II-2f)

Workout #3A

Butt and Lower Body & Stomach and Thighs

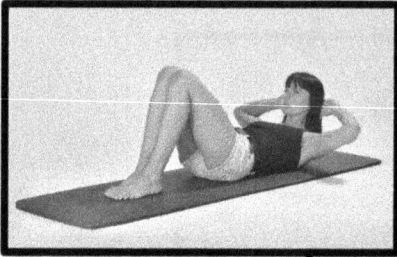

1

Standard Crunch
(S1-L II-2a)

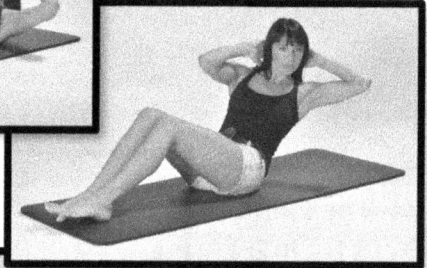

2

Standard
Crunch
(with
a twist)
(S1-L II-2b)

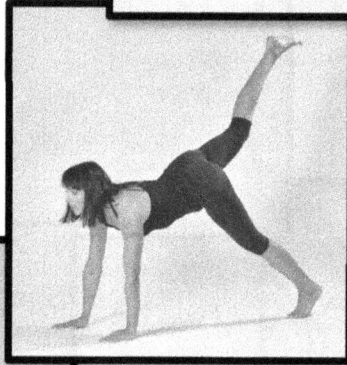

3

Backward
Leg-Lifts
(Version #2)
(S1-L II-1f)

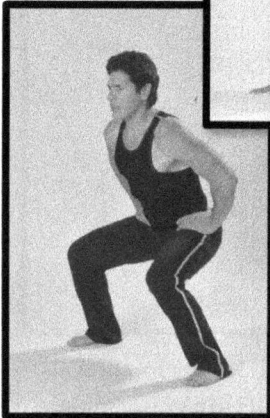

4

Standard Squats
(S1-L II-1a)

Workout #3B

Butt and Lower Body & Stomach and Thighs

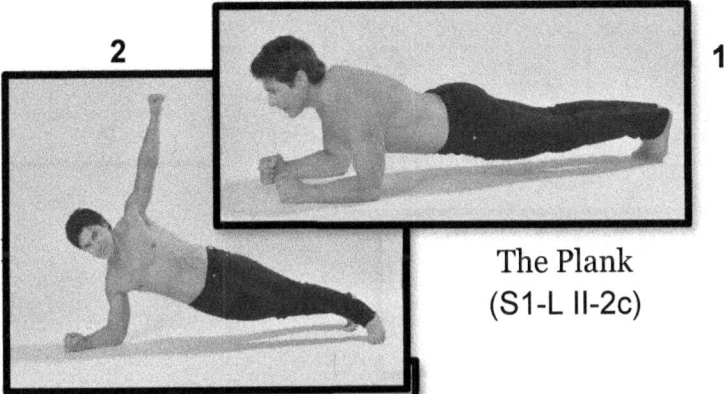

2

1

The Plank
(S1-L II-2c)

The
Twisting
Plank
(S1-L II-2d)

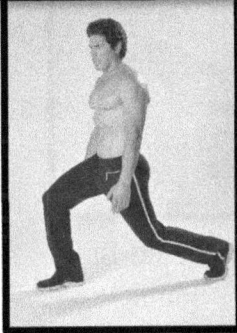

3

Standard
Lunges
(S1-L II-1d)

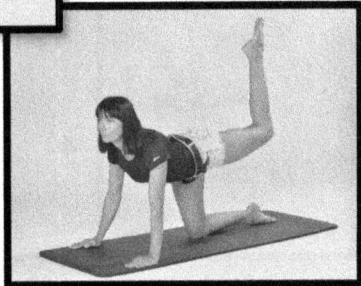

4

Backward Leg-Lifts
(Version #1) (S1-L II-1f)

Workout #3C

<u>Butt and Lower Body & Stomach and Thighs</u>

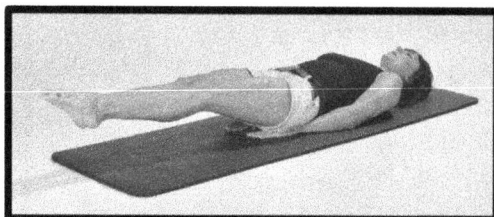

1

Forward Leg Lifts
(lying down)
(S1-L II-2e)

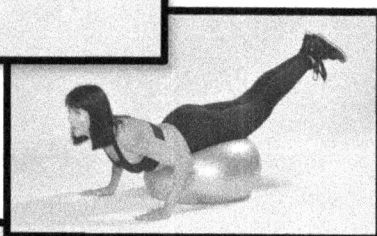

2

Medicine-Ball
Backward
Leg Lifts
(S1-L II-1g)

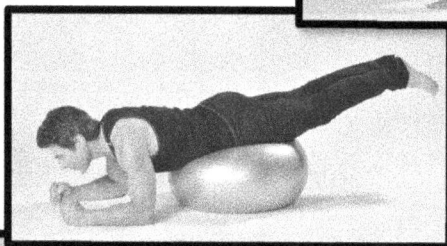

3

Medicine-Ball
Plank
(S1-L II-1h)

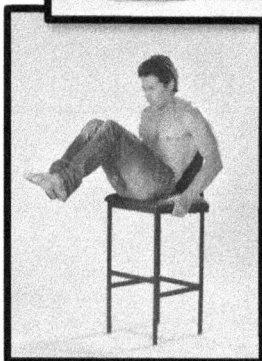

4

Forward Leg Lifts
(sitting) (Version #1)
(S1-L II-2f)

Workout #4A

Push-Ups & Curls, Lifts and Pushes

2

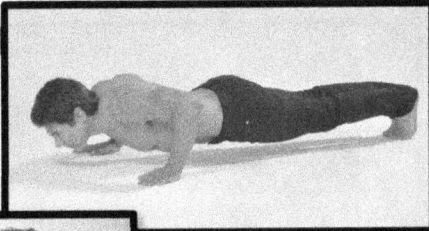

1

3

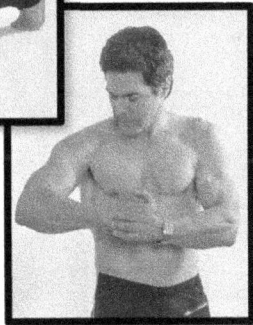

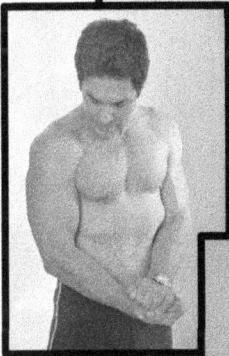

Standard
Push-Ups
(Version #1)
(S1-L II-3a)

Chest Push
(S1-L II-4g)

4

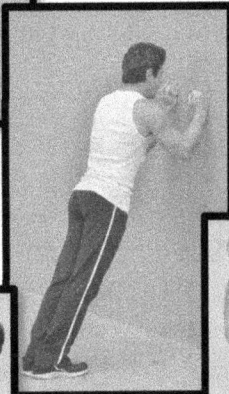

5

Freestyle
Curls
(S1-L II-4b)

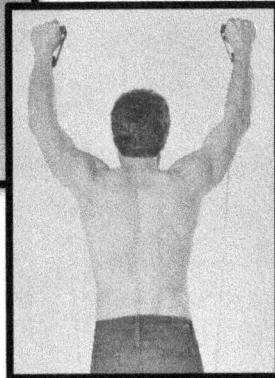

6

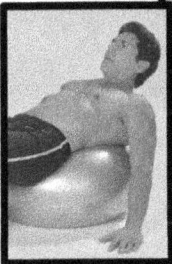

Triceps
Push
(S1-L II-4d)

Medicine-Ball
Neck Lifts
(S1-L II-4j)

Shoulders Lift (S1-L II-4h)

Workout #4B

<u>Push-Ups & Curls, Lifts and Pushes</u>

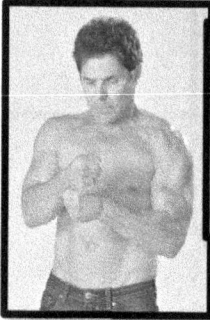

1

2

Standard Push-Ups
(Version #2)
(S1-L II-3a)

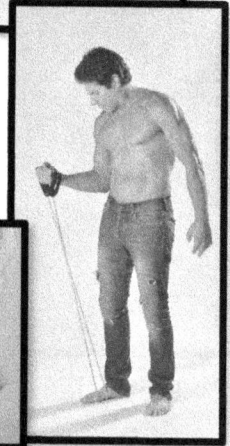

Chest
"Rope Pull"
(S1-L II-4f)

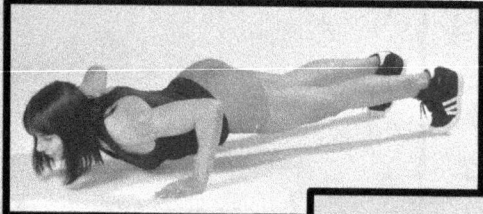

3

4

5

Forearm Push
(S1-L II-4e)

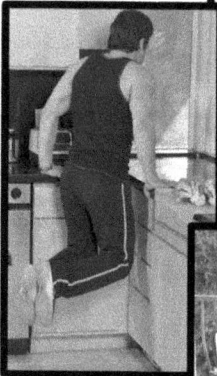

Band Curls
(S1-L II-4a)

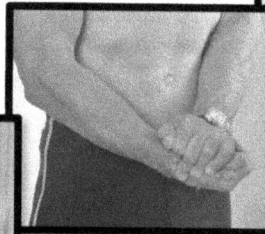

6

Triceps Push
(S1-L II-4d)

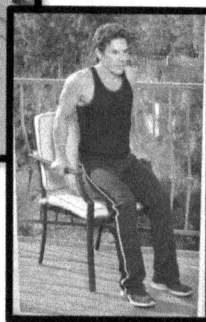

Moving Lats Lift (S1-L II-4i)

Workout #5A

Whole Body

2

1

3

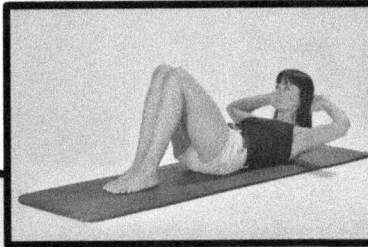

Standard Crunch
(S1-L II-2a)

4

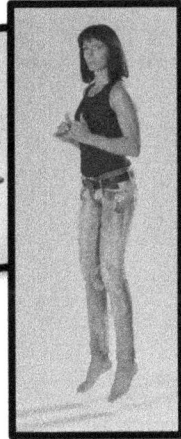

Basic
Hopping
(S1-L II-5a)

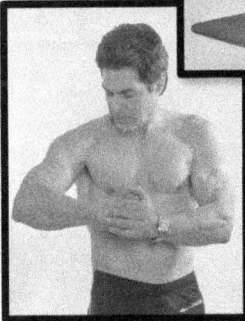

Chest Push
(S1-L II-4g)

7

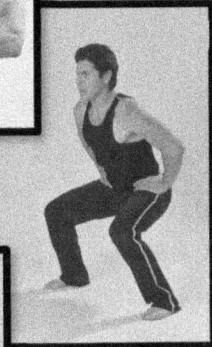

Standard
Squats
(S1-L II-1a)

5

6

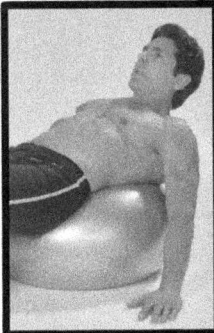

Medicine-Ball
Neck Lifts
(S1-L II-4j)

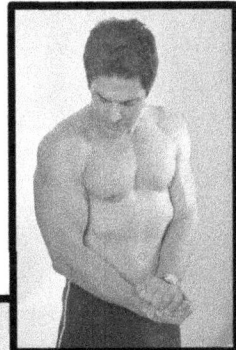

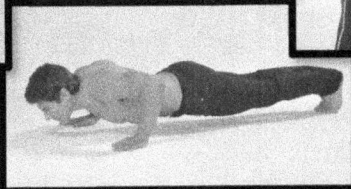

Freestyle
Curls
(S1-L II-4b)

Standard Push-Ups (Version #1) (S1-L II-3a)

Workout #5B

<u>Whole Body</u>

1

2

The Plank
(S1-L II-2c

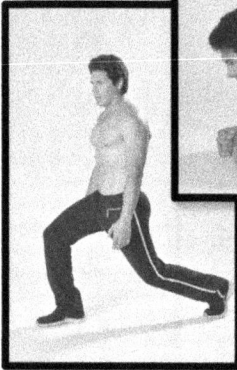

Standard
Lunges
(S1-L II-1d)

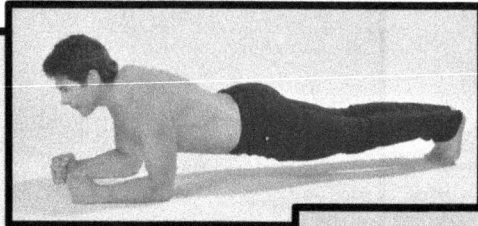

3

4

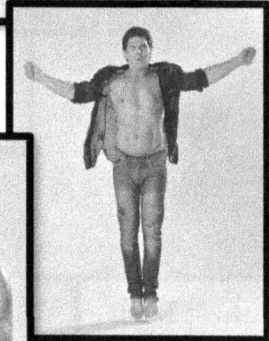

Imaginary
Jump Rope
(S1-L II-5b)

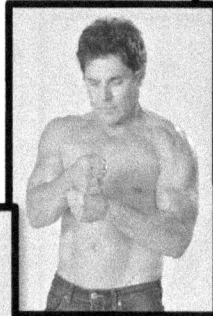

Chest
"Rope Pull"
(S1-L II-4f)

5

6

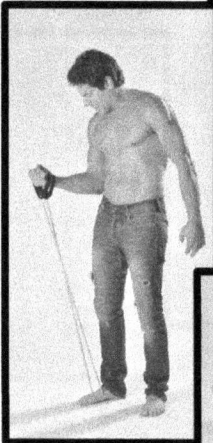

Band Curls
(S1-L II-4a)

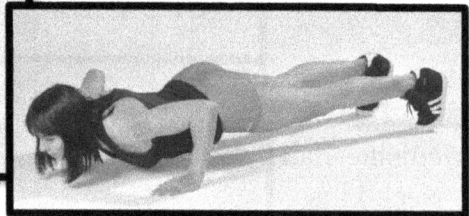

Standard Push-Ups
(Version #2) (S1-L II-3a)

Workout #5C

Whole Body

1

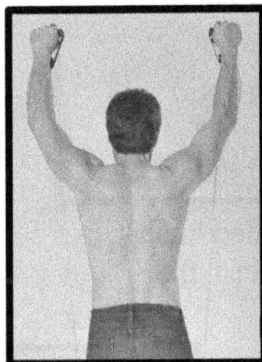

Shoulders Lift
(S1-L II-4h)

2

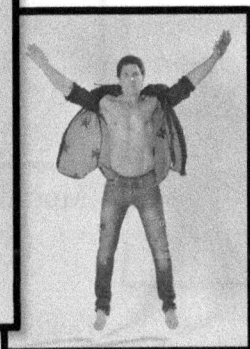

Jumping Jacks
(S1-L II-5c)

3

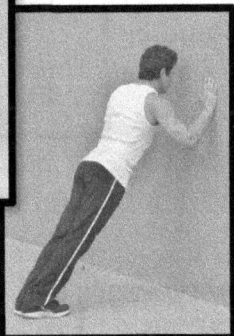

Angled
Push-Ups
(S1-L II-3b)

5

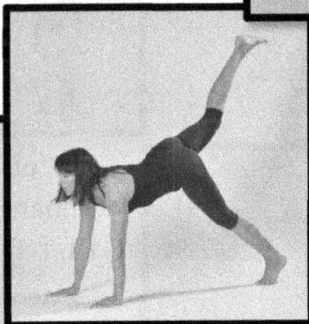

Forward Leg Lifts
(sitting)
(Version #2)
(S1-L II-2f)

4

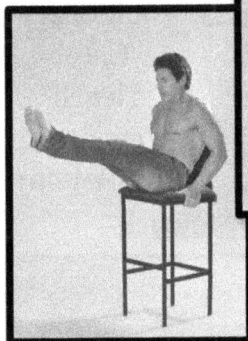

Backward
Leg Lifts
(Version #2)
(S1-L II-1f)

6

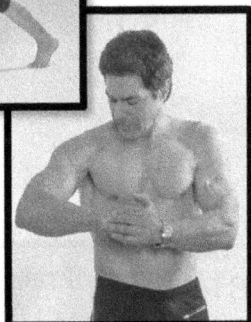

Chest Push
(S1-L II-4g)

Additions and Substitutions
(Part 1)

Butt

Chest/Triceps

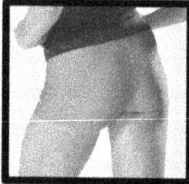

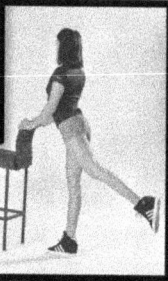

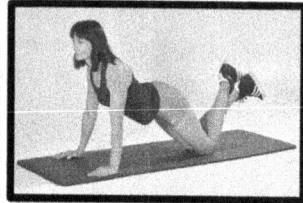

Standing
-Still
Butt
Clench*
(S1-L I-1a)

Standing
Butt Clench
Leg Lifts*
(balancing)
(S1-L I-1d)

Modified Push-Ups
(S1-L II-3c)

Chest

Biceps

Kegels

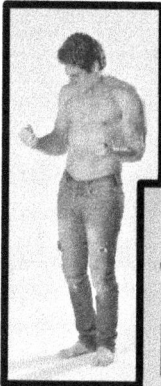

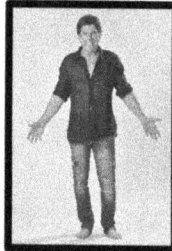

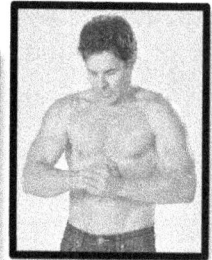

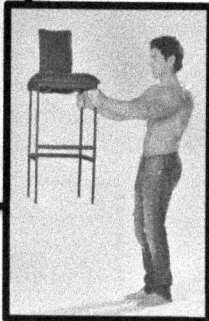

Kegel
Clench*
(S1-L I-11a)

Stationary
Chest
Clench*
(Version #2)
(S1-L I-4a)

Stomach

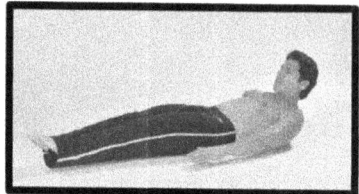

Curl
Clench
Pump*
(S1-L I-3a)

Freestyle
Lifts
(S1-L II-4c)

*mix in some clenches.

Stomach Clench Crunch*
(lying down) (S1-L I-2a)

Additions and Substitutions
(Part 2)

<u>Stretching</u>

Quad Stretch – 2
(S1-L II-6d)

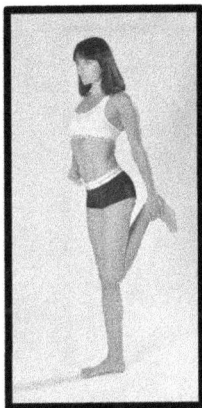

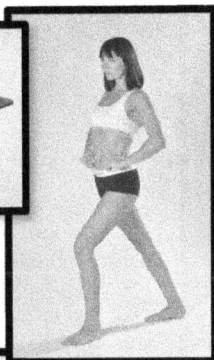

Quad
Stretch – 1
(S1-L II-6c)

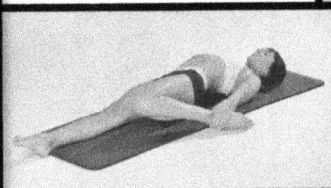

Glutes/Lower Back
Stretch (S1-L II-6a)

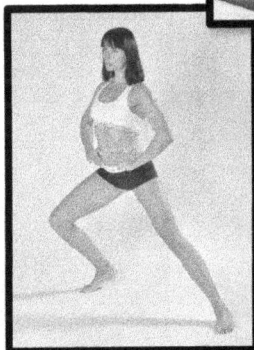

Calf
Stretch
(S1-L II-6f)

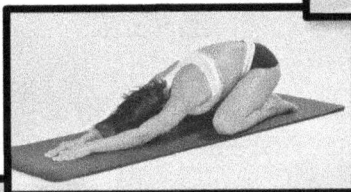

Inner Thigh
Stretch
(S1-L II-6e)

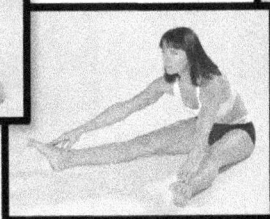

Hamstring
Stretch
(S1-L II-6b)

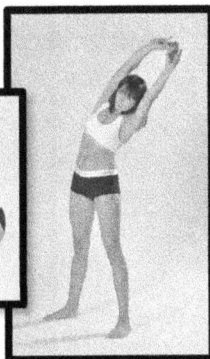

Obliques Stretch
(S1-L II-6h)

Additions and Substitutions
(Part 3)

<u>Stretching</u>

Forearm
Stretch – 1
(S1-L II-6k)

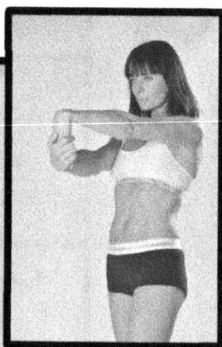

Forearm
Stretch – 2
(S1-L II-6l)

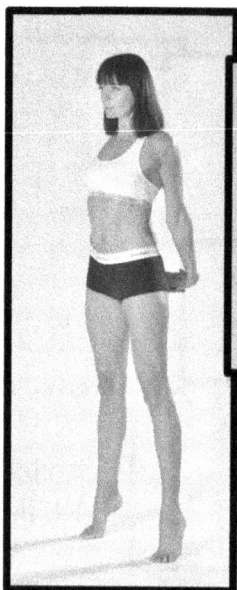

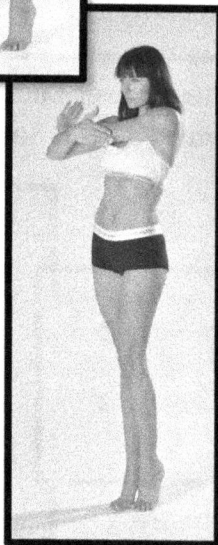

Chest
Stretch
(S1-L II-6j)

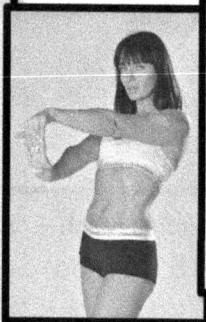

Triceps
Stretch
(S1-L II-6m)

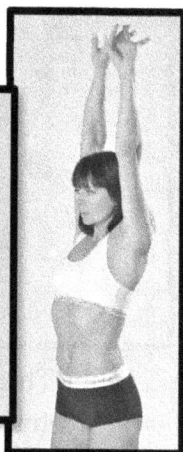

Lats/Biceps
Stretch
(S1-L II-6g)

Shoulder
Stretch (S1-L II-6i)

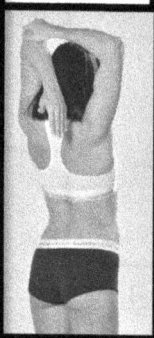

Additions and Substitutions
(Part 4)

Duo Stretching

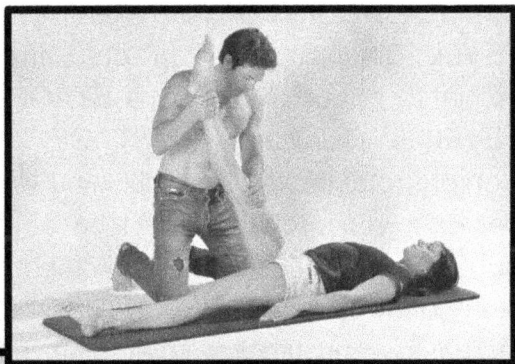

Duo Hamstring
Stretch
(S1-L II-7a)

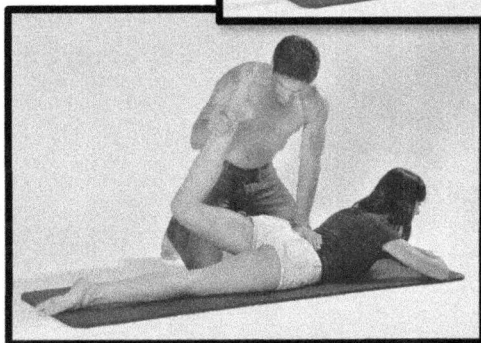

Duo Quad
Stretch
(S1-L II-7b)

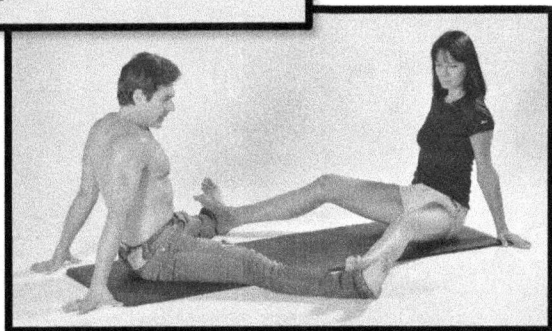

Duo Inner-Thigh/Butt Stretch (S1-L II-7c)

STAGE 4
(Advanced Exercise Routines)

These routines use the exercises from STAGE 1, LEVEL 3. Again, if you can arrange your time efficiently enough, add some STAGE 1, LEVEL I and LEVEL II exercises and STAGE 2 and STAGE 3 workout routines into the mix. And like STAGE 3, just because you probably won't be able to do them in public, is no excuse not to do them. Managing your time to do one of these routines daily will greatly increase your fitness level. But remember, these routines are simply suggestions. You can always do more.

Workout #1

<u>Butt</u>

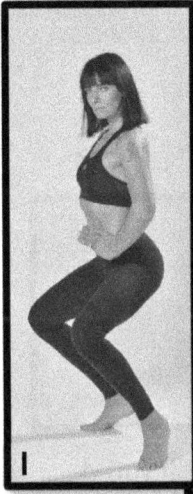
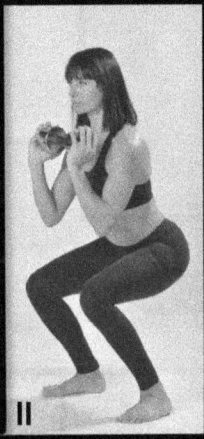
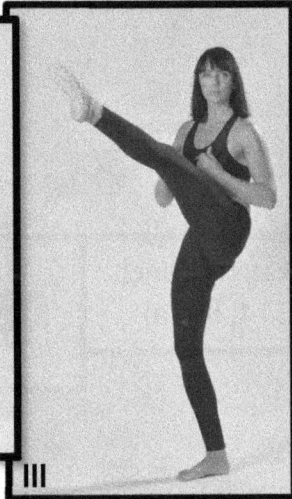

Triple Squats
(Parts I, II & III) (S1-L III-1d)

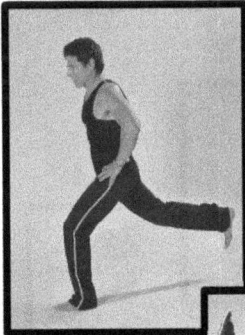
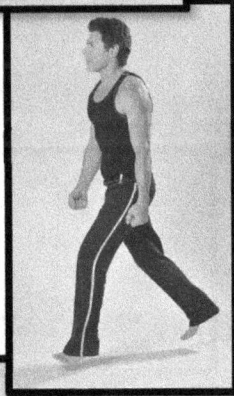
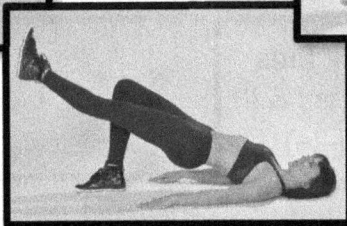

Lunge
Walking
(Version #2)
(S1-L III-1c)

Jumping
Lunges
(S1-L III-1b)

Bridge Butt Lifts (Version #2) (S1-L III-1d)

Workout #2

1   Stomach

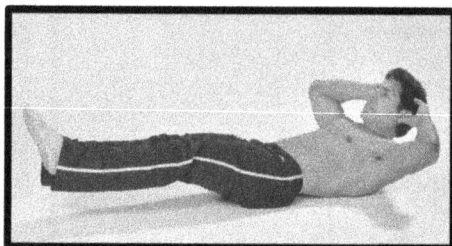

Elevated Crunch
(S1-L III-2a)

2

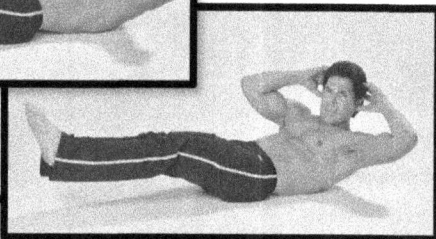

Elevated
Crunch
(with a twist)
(S1-L III-2b)

3

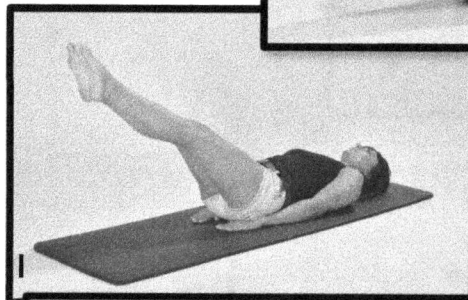

I

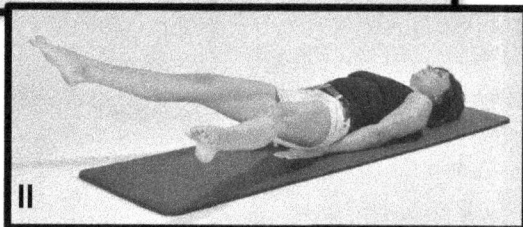

II

Scissor Leg Lifts
Combo (Parts I & II)
(S1-L III-2e)

4

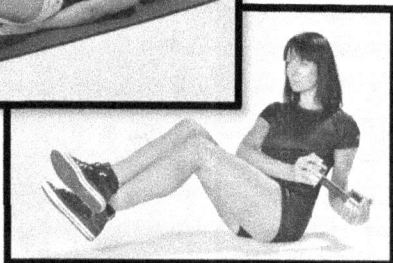

Elevated Twisting Crunch
(with weight) (S1-L III-2c)

Workout #3A

Butt and Stomach

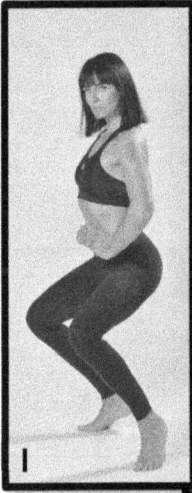

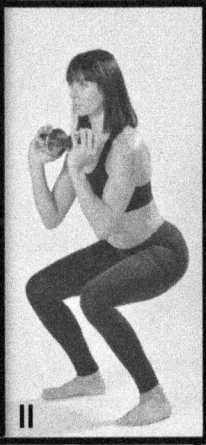

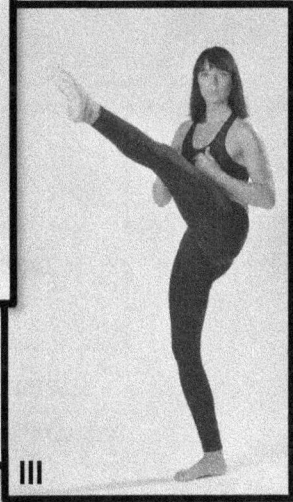

1

Triple Squats
(Parts I, II, & III)
(S1-L III-1d)

2

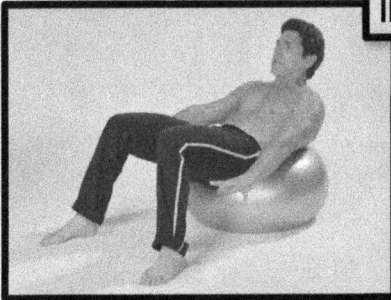

Medicine-Ball
Crunch
(S1-L III-2f)

3

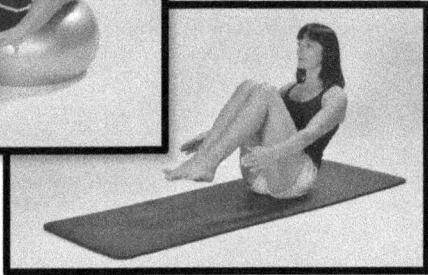

Folding Crunch (S1-L III-2d)

Workout #3B

Butt and Stomach

1

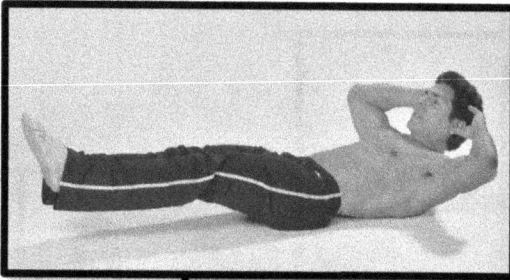

Elevated
Crunch
(S1-L III-2a)

2

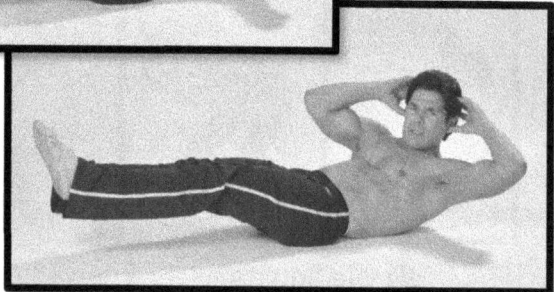

Elevated Crunch
(with a twist)
(S1-L III-2b)

4

3

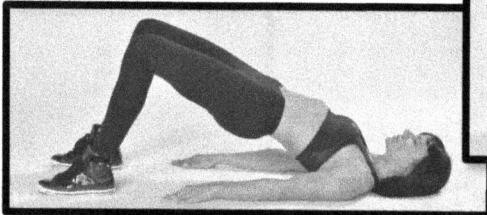

Bridge Butt Lifts
(Version #1) (S1-L III-1a)

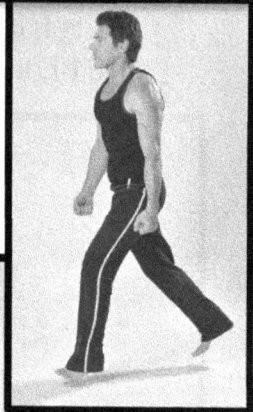

Jumping
Lunges
(S1-L III-1b)

Workout #3C

Butt and Stomach

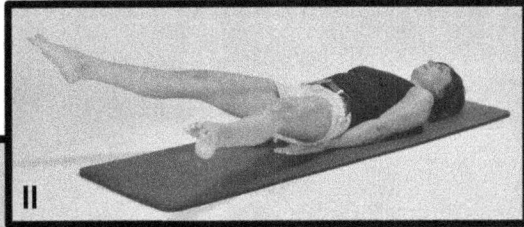

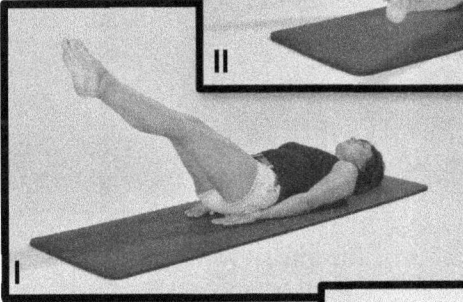

Scissor Leg Lifts
Combo
(Parts I & II)
(S1-L III-2e)

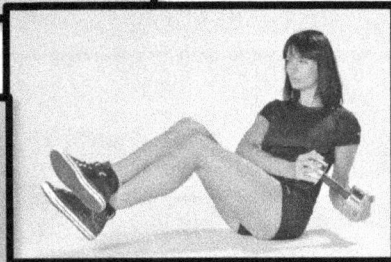

Elevated Twisting Crunch
(with weight) (S1-L III-2c)

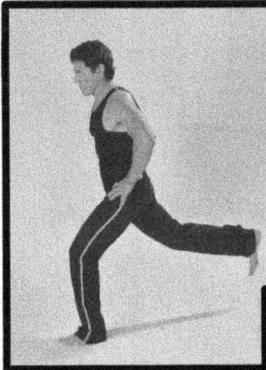

Lunge
Walking
(Version #2)
(S1-L III-1c)

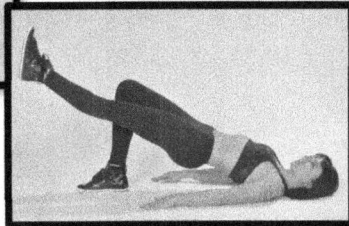

Bridge Butt Lifts
(Version #2) (S1-L III-1a)

Workout #4A

1 <u>Push-Ups, Upper Body and Chin-Up Bar</u>

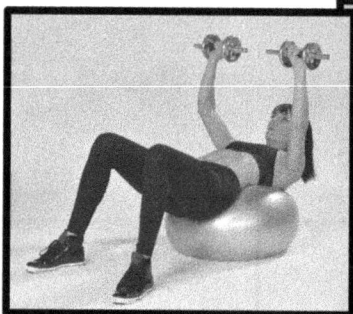

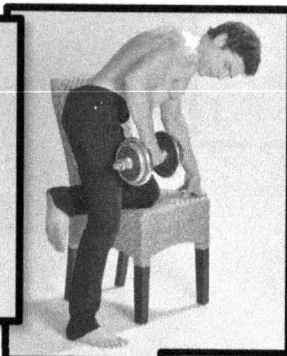

2

3

Medicine-Ball
Chest Press
(S1-L III-4b)

Lats Pull
(S1-L III-4g)

5

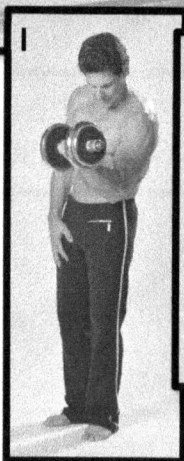

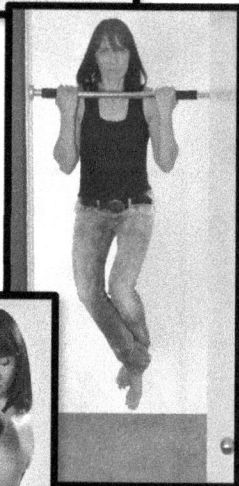

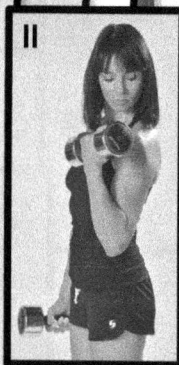

Advanced
Push-Ups
(Version #1)
(S1-L III-3a)

Standard
Pull-Ups
(S1-L III-5a)

4

Curls (Parts I & II) (S1-L III-4a)

Workout #4B

Push-Ups, Upper Body and Chin-Up Bar

1

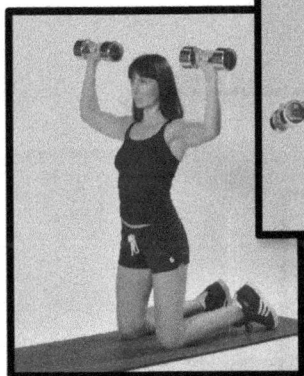

2

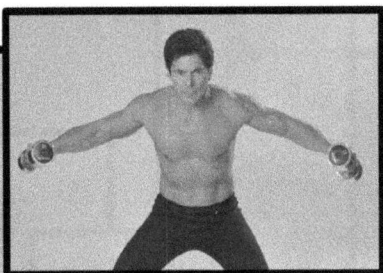

Backward Fly
(S1-L III-4f)

Shoulder
Press
(S1-L III-4d)

3

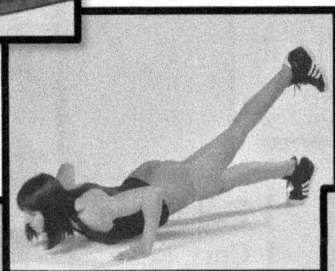

Push-Ups
(with
leg lifts)
(S1-L III-3c)

I

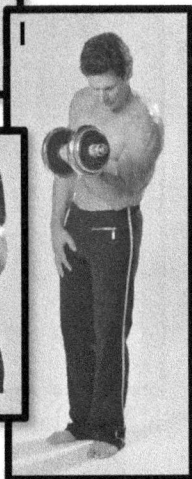

II

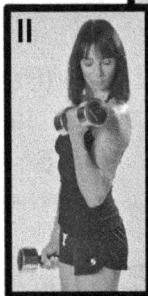

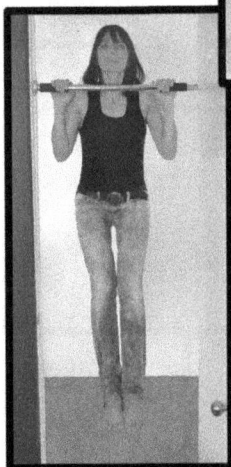

4

5

Standard Chin-Ups
(S1-L III-5b)

Curls (Parts I & II)
(S1-L III-4a)

Workout #4C

<u>Push-Ups, Upper Body and Chin-Up Bar</u>

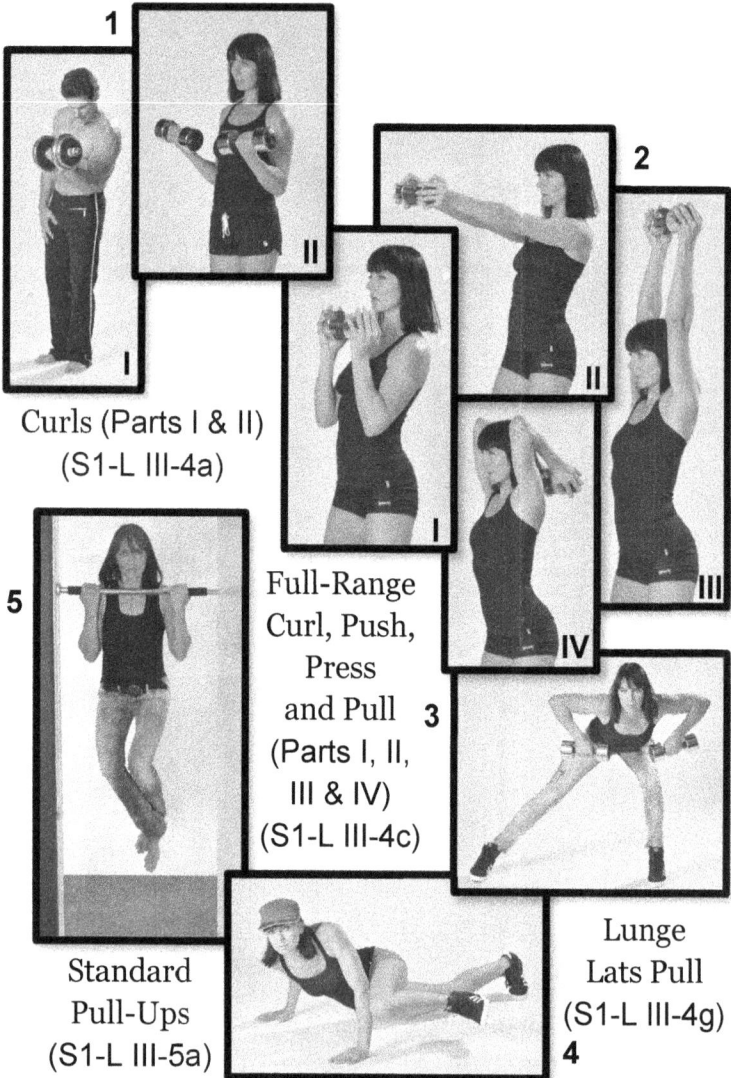

Curls (Parts I & II)
(S1-L III-4a)

Full-Range
Curl, Push,
Press
and Pull
(Parts I, II,
III & IV)
(S1-L III-4c)

Standard
Pull-Ups
(S1-L III-5a)

Lunge
Lats Pull
(S1-L III-4g)

Leg Crunch Push-Ups (Version #1) (S1-L III-3d)

Workout #5A (Part 1)

1

Whole Body

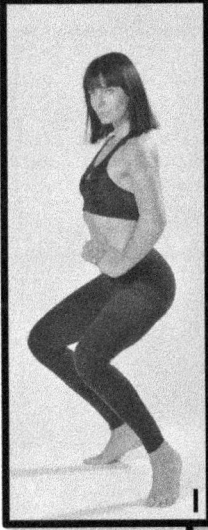

Triple
Squats
(Parts I, II
& III)
(S1-L III-1d)

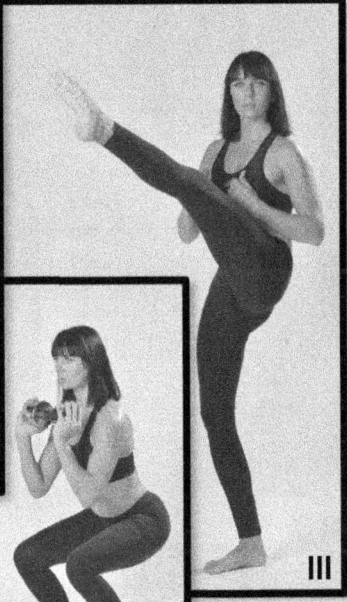

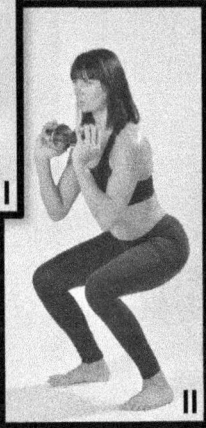

2

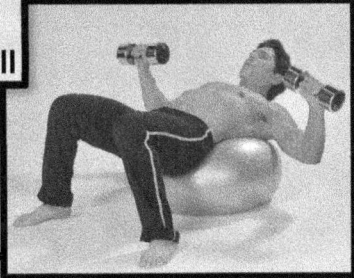

Medicine-Ball
Chest Press
(S1-L III-4b)

3

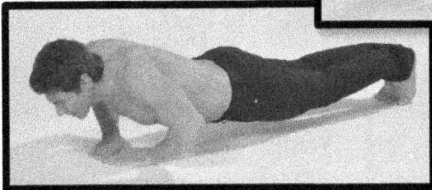

Advanced Push-Ups (Version #2) (S1-L III-3a)

Workout #5A (Part 2)

<u>Whole Body</u>

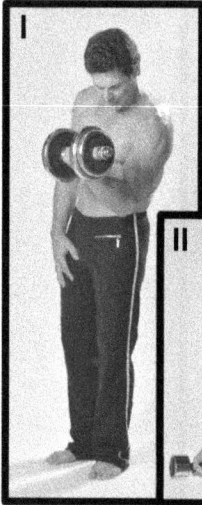

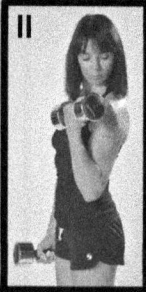

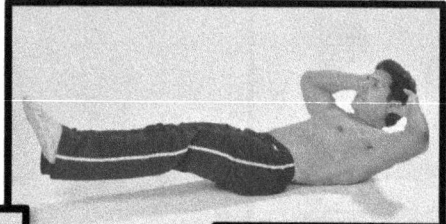

Elevated
Crunch
(S1-L III-2a)

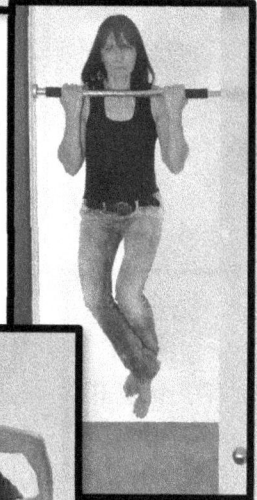

Curls (Parts I & II)
(S1-L III-4a)

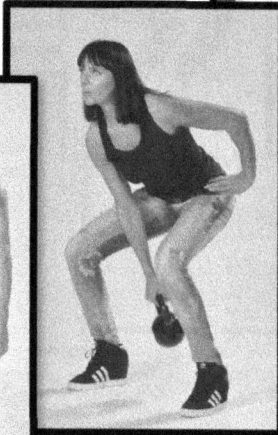

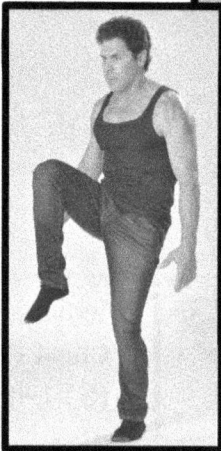

Standard
Pull-Ups
(S1-L III-5a)

Weight Swing
(S1-L III-6a)

Running in Place (S1-L III-7d)

Workout #5B (Part 1)

Whole Body

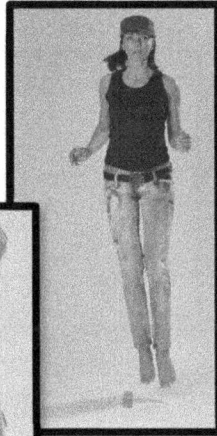

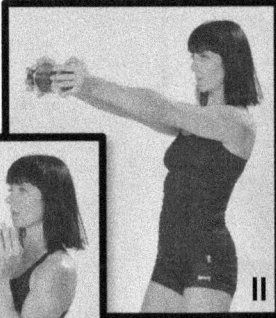

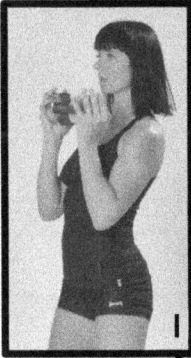

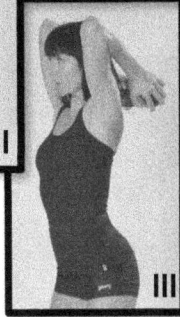

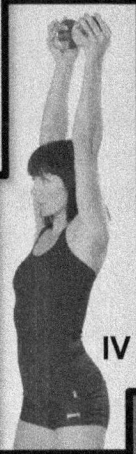

Precision
Jumping
(S1-L III-7a)

Full-Range
Curl, Push, Press and Pull
(Parts I, II, III & IV) (S1-L III-4c)

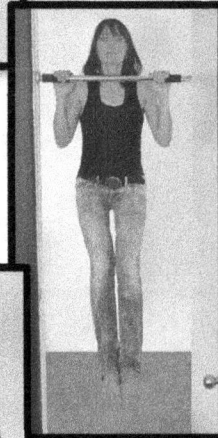

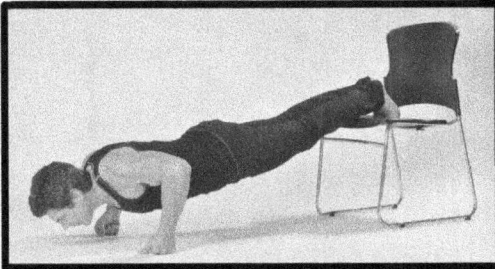

Standard
Chin-Ups
(S1-L III-5b)

Decline Push-Ups (S1-L III-3b)

Workout #5B (Part 2)

<u>Whole Body</u>

5

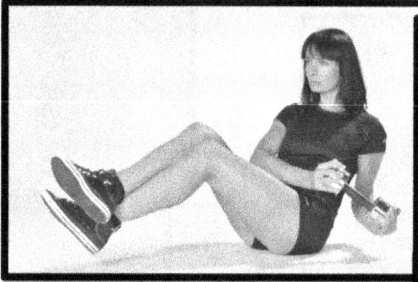

Elevated Twisting Crunch
(with weight) (S1-L III-2c)

6

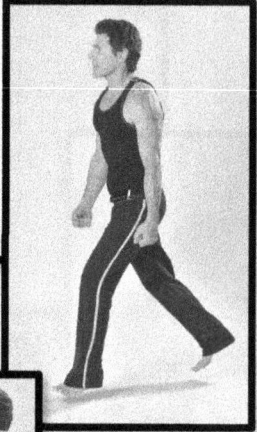

Jumping
Lunges
(S1-L III-1b)

7

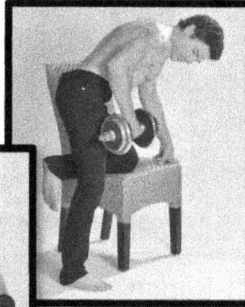

Lats Pull
(S1-L III-4g)

8

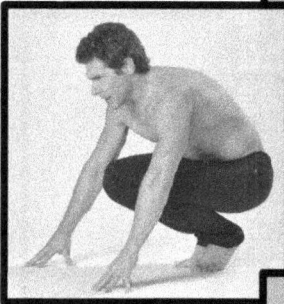

Burpees
(S1-L III-6b)

9

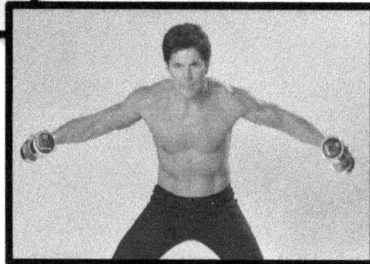

Backward Fly (S1-L III-4f)

Workout #5C (Part 1)

1

<u>Whole Body</u>

2

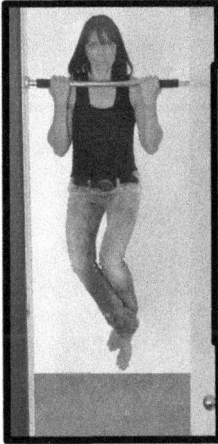

Standard
Pull-Ups
(S1-L III-5a)

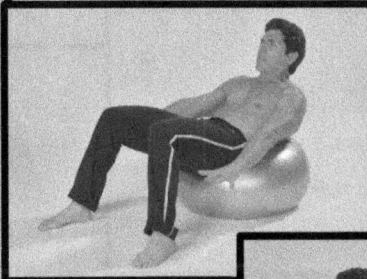

Medicine-Ball
Crunches
(S1-L III-2f)

3

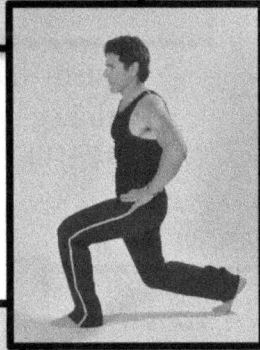

Lunge Walking
(Version #1)
(S1-L III-1c)

4

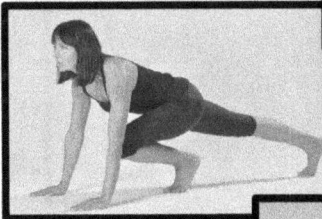

Mountain Climb
(S1-L III-6c)

5

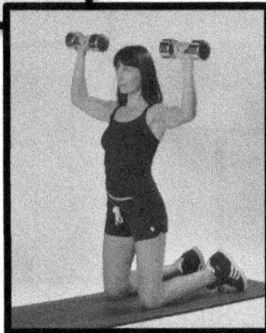

Shoulder Press (S1-L III-4d)

Workout #5C (Part 2)

<u>Whole Body</u>

6

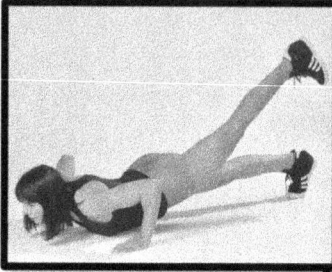

Push-Ups
with Leg Lifts
(S1-L III-3c)

7

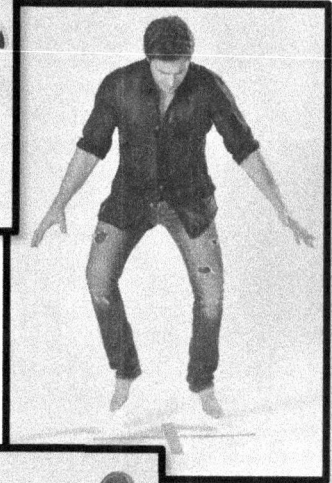

Precision
Hopping
(S1-L III-7b)

8

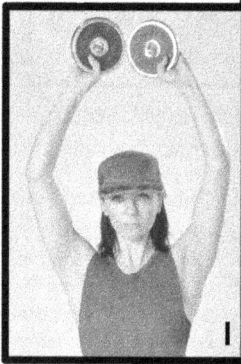

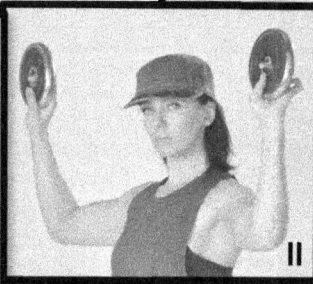

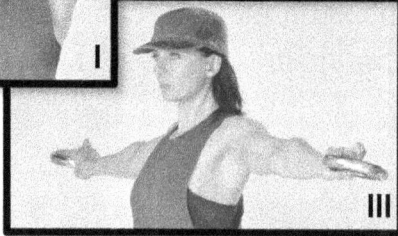

Shoulder Swings (with weights)
(Parts I, II & III) (S1-L III-4e)

Workout #5D (Part 1)

Whole Body

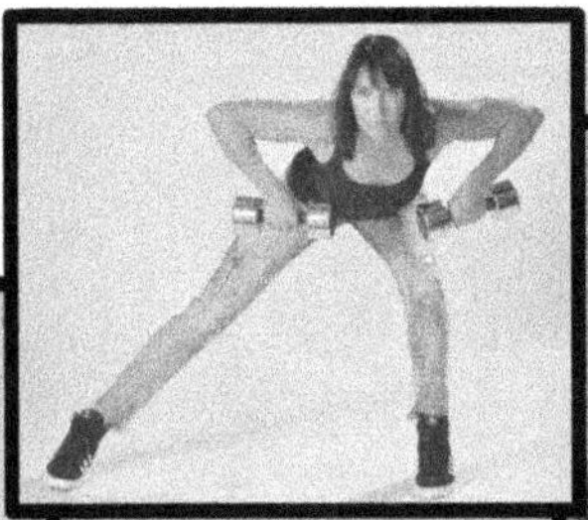

**Lunge Lats Pull
(S1-L III-4h)**

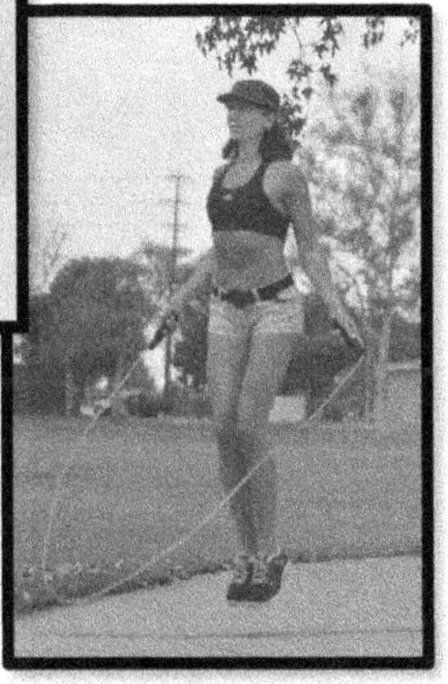

**Jumping Rope
(S1-L III-7c)**

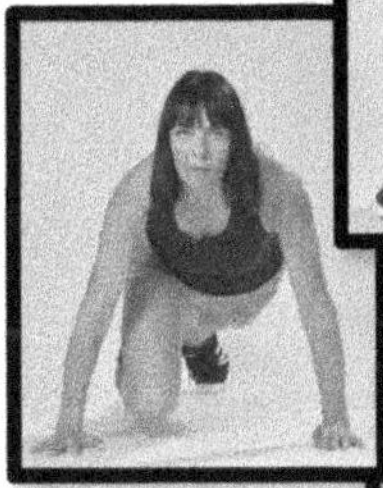

Leg Crunch
Push-Ups
(Version #2)
(S1-L III-7c)

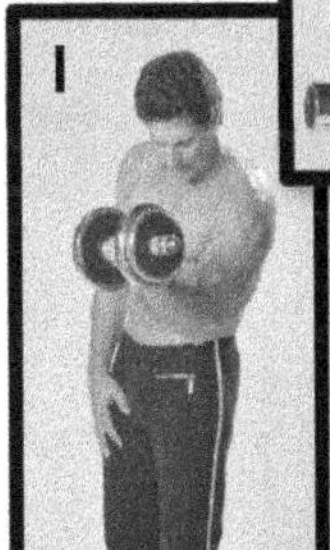

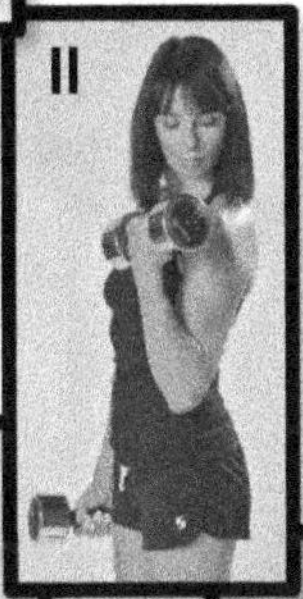

Curls
(Parts I & II)
(S1-L III-4a)

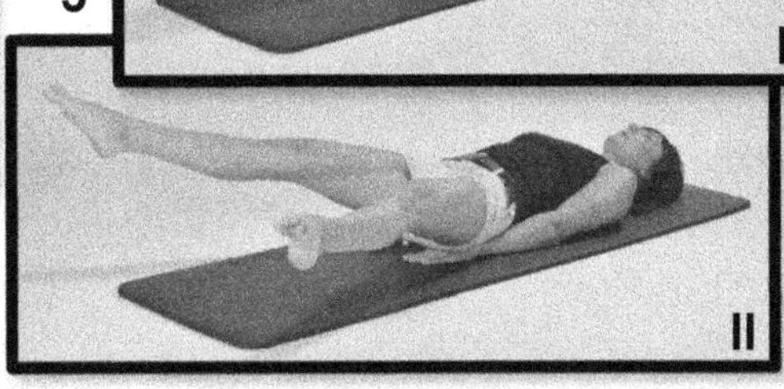

Scissor Leg Lifts Combo (Parts I & II) (S1-L III-2e)

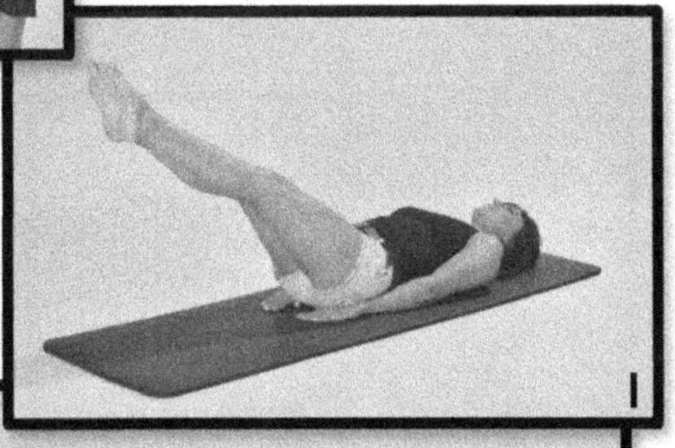

Workout #5D (Part 2)

Whole Body

6

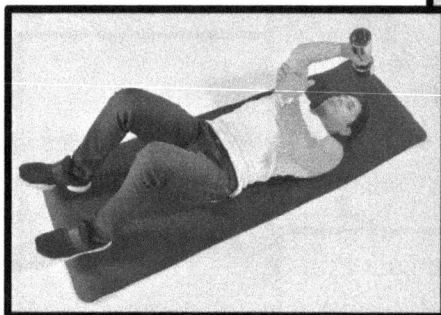

Triceps Press (w/weight)
(with support) (S1-L III-4j)

7

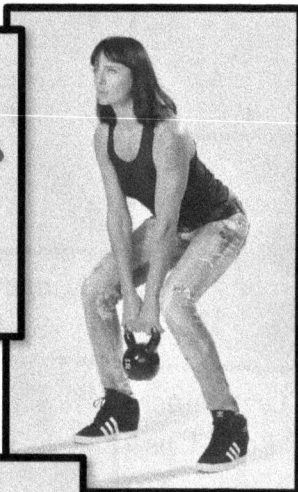

Weight Swing
(S1-L III-6a)

8

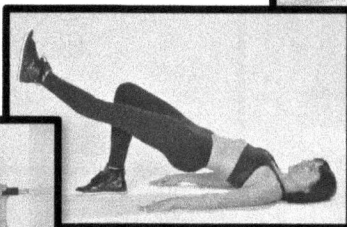

Bridge
Butt Lifts
(Version #2)
(S1-L III-1a)

9

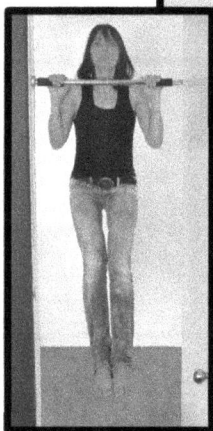

Standard
Chin-Ups
(S1-L III-5b)

10

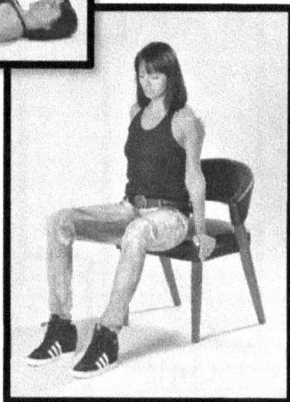

Sitting Hip Abductor
(S1-L III-1g)

Extra Credit (Part 1)

Stomach

Pull-Ups & Chin-Ups

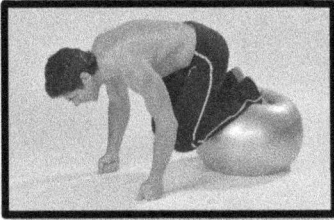

Medicine-Ball Leg Rolls
(S1-L III-2g)

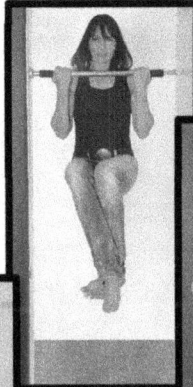

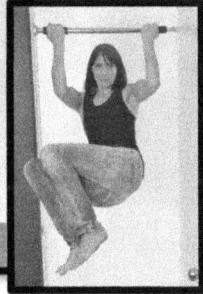

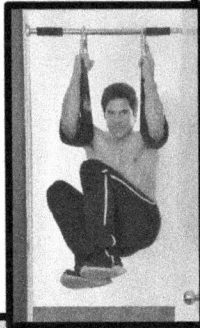

Leg Lift
Pull-Ups
(Versions
#1 & #2)
(S1-L III-5d)

Leg Lift
Pull-Ups
(Versions
#3 & #4)
(S1-L III-5d)

Chin-Up
Bar
Leg Lifts
(Version #2)
(S1-L III-5c)

Butt

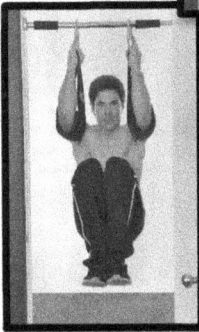

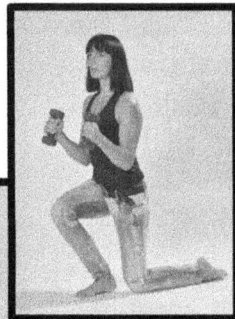

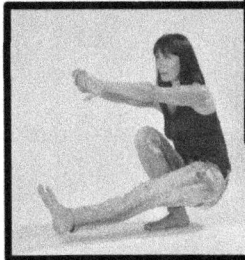

Chin-Up Bar
Leg Lifts
(Version #1)
(S1-L III-5c)

Extended Leg
Floor Squat
(S1-L III-1e)

Single-Leg Lunges (with weights) (S1-L III-1f)

Extra Credit (Part 2)

Full Body

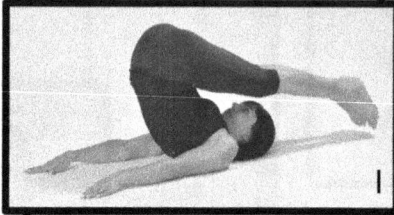

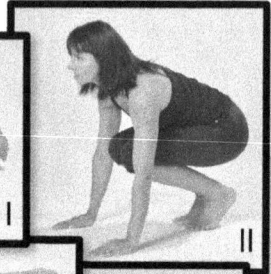

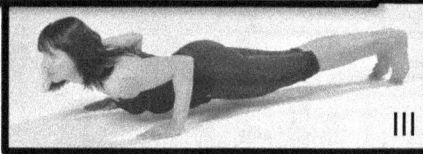

Lift, Roll, Push and Jump
(Parts I, II, III & IV)
(S1-L III-6d)

Push-Ups

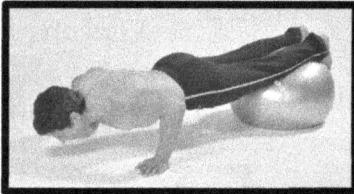

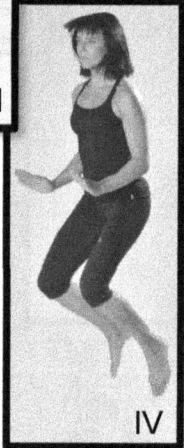

Medicine-Ball
Push-Ups
(S1-L III-3e)

Aerobics

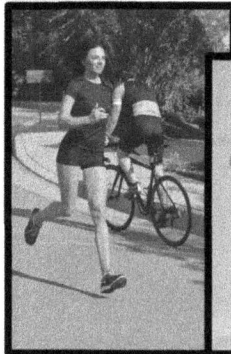

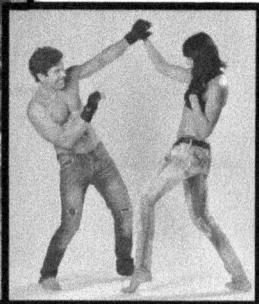

Running (fast) – Cycling (distance)
– Sports (challenge) (S1-L III-7e)

Additions and Substitutions (Part 1)

Butt

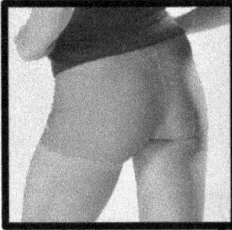

Standing Still
Butt Clench*
(S1-L I-1a)

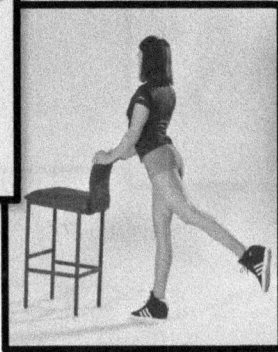

Standing
Butt Clench
Leg Lifts*
(balancing)
(S1-L I-1d)

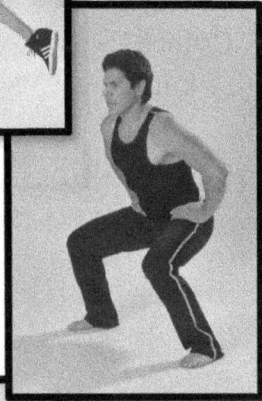

Standard
Squats*
(S1-L I-1a)

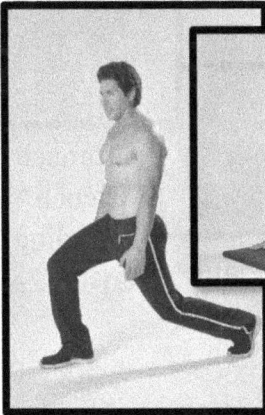

Standard Lunges*
(S1-L II-1e)

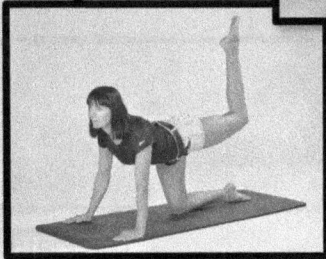

Backward
Leg Lifts
(Version #1)*
(S1-L II-1f)

Additions and Substitutions (Part 2)

<u>Stomach</u>

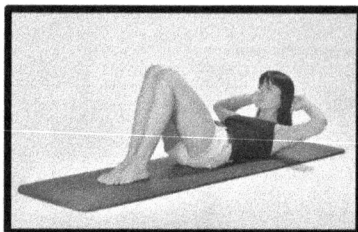

Standard
Crunch*
(S1-L II-2a)

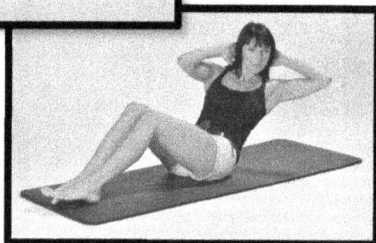

Standard Crunch*
(with a twist)
(S1-L II-2b)

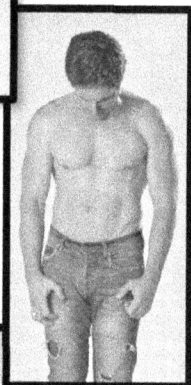

Stomach
Clench*
(Standing)
(S1-L I-2a)

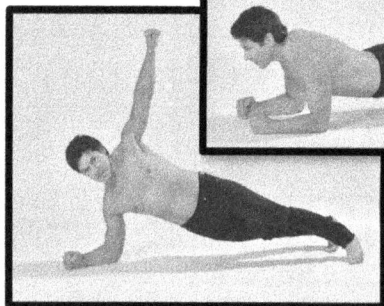

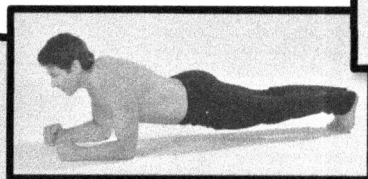

The Plank*
(S1-L II-2c)

The Twisting Plank*
(S1-L II-2d)

Additions and Substitutions (Part 3)

Arms and Chest

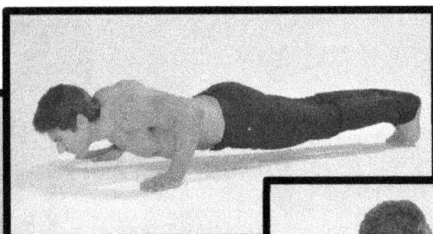

Standard
Push-Ups*
(Version #1)
(S1-L II-3a)

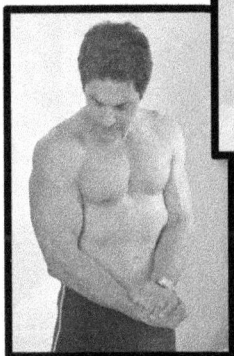

Freestyle
Curls*
(S1-L II-4b)

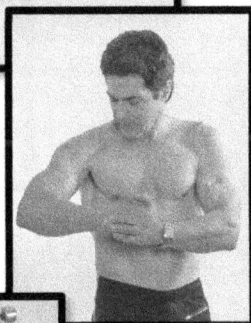

Chest Push*
(S1-L II-4g)

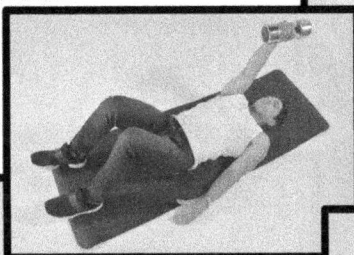

Triceps Press
(with weight)
(without
support)
(S1-L III-4j)

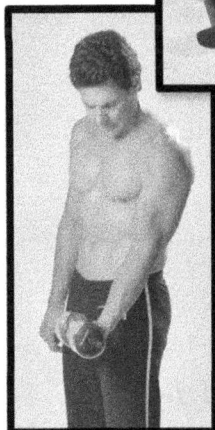

Chest
"Rope Pull"*
(S1-L II-4f)

Forearm Lifts
(S1-L III-4i)

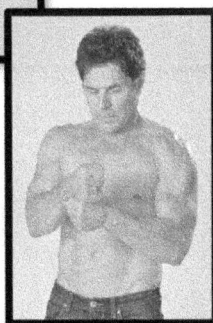

Additions and Substitutions (Part 4)

Misc. Exercises

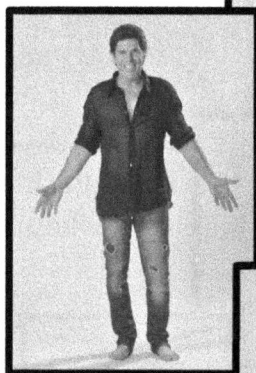

Jumping Jacks*
(S1-L II-5c)

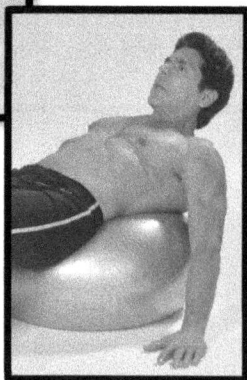

Calves Lift
(S1-L III-1h)

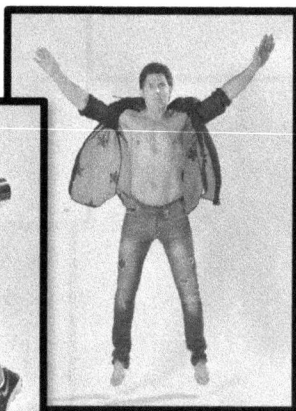

Kegel
Clench*
(S1-L I-11a)

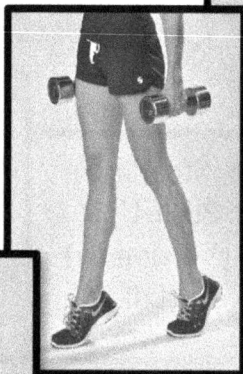

Medicine-Ball Neck Lifts (S1-L II-4j)*

*Try adding some Clenches and Level II exercises, too.

Additions and Substitutions (Part 5)

Duo Exercises

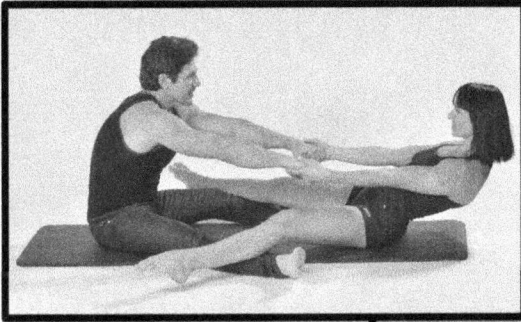

Duo See-Saw
(S1-L III-8c)

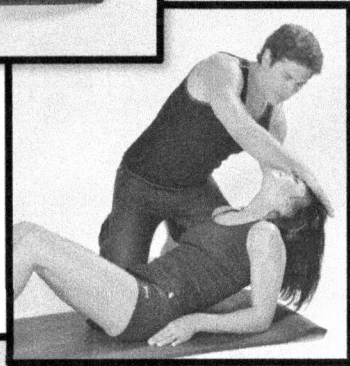

Duo
Neck
Lifts
(S1-L III-8a)

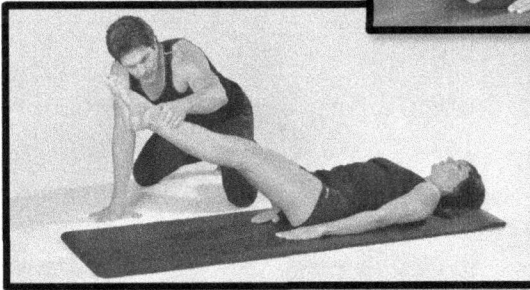

Duo Upper-Leg Lifts
(S1-L III-8b)

– Section 3 –

Xer-tasking for life

(incentives and tips to keep you going)

"Effort only fully releases its reward after a person refuses to quit." – Napoleon Hill

5   THE MOTIVATION OF GUILT

"Even I don't always want to exercise. So, I installed a chin-up bar between the sides of a door frame that I walk through a lot. That way I'm forced to see it. And if I pass under it too many times without using it I start to feel guilty. And I swear at myself. 'You lazy...' When I feel guilty enough, I do a set. I'm not a big believer in letting guilt rule my life. But in the case of exercising and eating right, if that's what it takes, then I'm all for it. In fact, if you aren't exercising in some way, no matter how small, then you should feel guilty. Exercise by guilt. It's a Hell of a way to do it. But if it works, I say do it, you lazy..." – Billy

Using a chin-up bar can work your forearms, triceps, biceps, lats, abs, glutes and quads. And if installed in a doorway, every time you pass under that bar you will be aware that you should be doing something to get and keep in shape. You might even use it. Maybe just seeing the bar will remind you to eat a little healthier. Or maybe it will remind you to take a longer walk. Or maybe you will do an exercise or two that you might not otherwise have done. See? The chin-up bar is a better piece of equipment than you thought. Just looking at it can make you sweat.

What works for the chin-up bar is also a good little trick for weights as well. You don't need a full rack of dumbbells but two sets of different poundage (i.e. 5/10; 10/15; 15/20) or at least one set of tens is something you might consider having. In fact, most people already do... somewhere. They keep them in places like under the bed, in the closet, or up in the attic collecting dust because "someday" they plan on using them. From our experience, unless you have something or someone to push you into it, "someday" may never come.

So, try this. If you don't have a couple weights, get some. Put them somewhere where you will have to see them; somewhere you'll see them before your little toe makes contact; somewhere it's easy to pick them up and do a few reps; or at least, somewhere you will see them so much that if you don't do some sort of exercise, or do something to improve your overall fitness, you will feel extremely guilty. If that doesn't work, then move the weights to a spot where you will absolutely catch your innocent feet. If that doesn't make you remember to exercise, then you deserve to crunch your little toe. And then you'll be forced to do one last meager exercise as you shove the weights under the bed, right next to the other set of weights that you forgot you had. Maybe the double guilt will have an effect. Maybe just the image of those weights lying beneath your underworked and over-fed body will get you started. Maybe not. But try. For your health's sake, try something.

Try leaving this book out in plain sight for you and everyone to see. Every time you look at it, the title will jump out at you. There it is: The Zero-Minute Workout. Can you honestly say you don't have zero-minutes to work out? One of the reasons you even considered any of this was probably because you said you had no time (zero-minutes) to workout. So, you already have all the time we require: Zero minutes! Is the guilt setting in yet?

Visiting friends and family will see the book and they will ask you about it, "What's this?" And what are you going to say?

"Oh that. It's a workout program that I don't have time for."

And they might ask, "How could you not have time for zero minutes? Everybody has that."

The guilt will be thrown your way from everywhere. Because the fact is, The Zero-Minute Workout requires only two things from you: 1) the very thing you probably claimed you had in the first place – no time; and 2) effort. And that's why we are making all the attempts to get you started and to keep you going. You need to make the effort. And if it takes a little guilt to get you to make better choices for your life, then so be it. In the long run – or walk – you'll be glad you finally did.

"Vitality shows in not only the ability to persist but the ability to start over."
– F. Scott Fitzgerald

6   RAMP THINGS UP A LITTLE

The Zero-Minute Workout will not ask more of you than you can do, so you shouldn't either. That being said, what is it that's stopping you from trying just a little bit harder? Most times, when we feel like we've gone as far as we can go or think we are giving things our all, truth is, that's not the truth. We can usually do quite a bit more. But all we are suggesting is a little bit more. And if you can do that, if you can increase your energy level just a little bit, that extra effort can go a long way to increasing the effectiveness of the results.

So, after you have done an exercise or an exercise routine for a while over several days or weeks, try ramping things up a little. Try to do those ten push-ups a little faster, then a little faster and a little faster still. Studies have found that a brisk ten-minute workout, twice a day, is more effective than a moderate twenty-minute workout once a day. We aren't saying that you should over-exert yourself, just suggesting that you might want to really give it your all, or close to it. It utilizes less of your time now and in the long run, the faster you see results the more apt you are to continue exercising. And that's the idea. Exercising is a life process, not just for now. Being fit is for always.

If you are going for a walk, then walk a little faster. Next time you are walking anywhere, notice the speed of your steps, the gate of your walk. Are you sauntering? Are you walking as if it doesn't matter how long it takes you to get to where you're going? If your answers are, yes, then pick up your pace. If you are unconsciously walking slow and listless, then consciously walk with renewed energy and purpose. Walk with a mission – the mission to get fit. And if you are out for a particularly long walk, you might want to consider doing it with a Walking Butt Clench or Lunge Walking or jogging or running part of the way. After a while, you might find it invigorating. You might even want to do it again... and again.

Next time you are presented with taking an elevator to your destination, try taking the stairs instead. Anything five floors or less is a good challenge that shouldn't be passed up. Walking upstairs is great for the butt and if the reason you were thinking of taking the elevator in the first place was to get to your desk and sit, all the more reason to walk up now. But don't stop there. If you can take two steps at a time, do that. And if you can run up the stairs, go for it. Five flights isn't really that far and the more you do it the more you'll be ready to tackle six flights and beyond. Use the railing to pull yourself along as your feet fly up the steps and you'll be amazed at the workout you'll get, all before you've even started your day at your desk.

Most big cities have some form of public transportation, but if you can, avoid it. And if that makes you feel guilty about taking money away from the city, then give a donation. Your energies are needed elsewhere. Pretend there are no buses or subways or cabs or Ubers or Lyfts and walk. Five, ten, twenty blocks can work wonders for your health and fitness, not to mention in some cities it may even be faster. And if riding a bike is safe enough, you might want to try it. It's a fun, super workout that gives you a great sense of accomplishment. Plus, it's good for the quality of air we all breathe and it's simply good for the quality of our lungs. Any time you can ride a bike, walk, run, hop, skip or jump your way to your destination instead of taking another mode of transportation, then do it. After a while it will become second nature and good for nature as well.

Unfortunately, for most people, it's normal to want to relax. For many of us, we claim we don't have time to relax any more than we have time to exercise. The more likely truth is somewhere in the middle. In actuality, you probably have the time to do whatever you choose to do. So, make what you choose to do, matter. If you need to relax, then do it. If you need to work, then do that. But if you don't need to relax or work and your time is not required of you elsewhere, then why not use the time for an X**er-task**? Why not defy the natural tendency to sit down and stop? You can sit, but don't stop.

Whenever you find yourself involved in an activity that doesn't require your full attention or can at least spare a second thought, then use that time for an exercise that turns those moments into **Xer-tasks.** The stomach, butt, chest, lats and legs can often be engaged or clenched without inhibiting your current activity and be unnoticed by those around you. So engage them! Clench them! It takes concerted effort, but the results are worth it. Your health will improve and the idea of exercising throughout the day will become habit. If you're walking the dog, walking from one desk to another, walking anywhere, stirring a pot at the stove, sitting down, lying down or just plain standing around you can easily turn your activity or inactivity into an **Xer-task.** And if you can do that consistently then you've managed to accomplish what The Zero-Minute Workout is all about.

The whole idea of life is to move forward; to keep going. Why not do it with the energy and vitality that comes from being in shape, at whatever biological age you find yourself being. Youth may be a time-based factor, but youthfulness doesn't have to be. And if you can keep exercising and not give up, you should find that youthfulness will be your norm, just as it should be. In other words, whatever activity you are doing, do it with gusto. And if it's worthwhile, then at the very least, it's worthwhile to try to do a little more.

"Make use of time, let not advantage slip."
– William Shakespeare

7   TIPS FOR FINDING TIME

You may still claim that you don't have any time to spare and maybe you don't. But chances are you do and we're willing to bet that you definitely have time to share or swap for an **Xer-task**. It may take some very creative time management on your part. It all depends on how serious you are about exercising. Following are a few suggestions on where to look.

1) Record a movie or TV show you want to see, instead of watching it when it's broadcast. An hour program could yield more than 20 minutes from commercials you probably don't want to see anyway.

2) Speaking of TV, just watching most 30-minute programs should yield three to five two-minute-plus blocks of time during the commercials that, again, it's a good bet you don't want to see.

3) Sticking with TV, when there is nothing on that you really want to watch, stop watching it! You could use the time for something else like... an exercise, or a whole exercise routine.

4) And lastly with TV, many programs don't require you to actually watch the screen, such as the news, talk shows and frankly, most broadcasts currently airing. Listening is enough. So, do an exercise along with it.

5) If you're spending too much time browsing social media, yet still can't break away, then try adding an Xer-task to your "addiction".

6) If you don't live alone, chances are from time to time you'll find yourself waiting to use the bathroom. Though you probably can't plan on this, you could have a list of exercises that you might do during such occasions. A Butt Clench comes to mind. In fact you may already be doing a Kegel without even thinking about it.

7) Speaking of clenching, it's a great idea to always have several clenches on your standby list for all the waiting time that life throws our way (i.e. banks, grocery stores, the DMV, traffic jams, etc.).

8) Make a list of all the Xer-tasking opportunities that are likely to come your way each day and be prepared to utilize them.

Keeping fit isn't an afterthought, it's a life-long planned activity. And before you know it, exercising and healthy living will simply become second nature.

"I spent my childhood eating. The only exercise I got was trying to twist off the cap of a jar of mayonnaise." – Richard Simmons

8   THINGS WE EAT

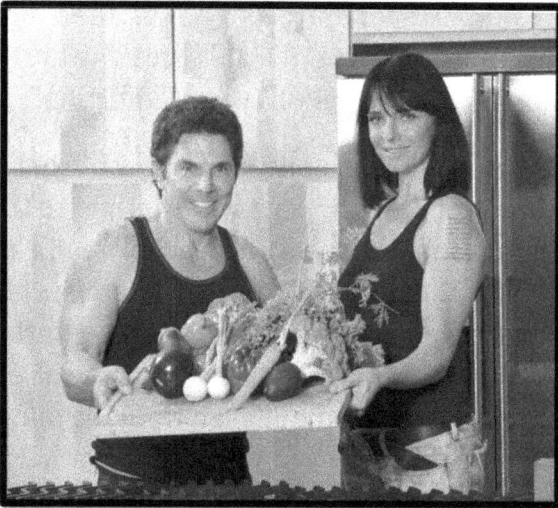

Most people eat by habit, not by what's best for them to eat or when the best time is to do it. They let their senses decide. And that's so often the problem.

"The smell of fresh bread is incredible. I grew up with it. My mother constantly made it. My father always had it in his car on the way to his restaurant. It was everywhere. But just because fresh, warm bread is so comforting, should I eat it? Hell no! Bread is like a floury siren calling us to certain, overweight, carb disaster. It still smells amazing. But I don't eat it. Ever." – Billy

This chapter gives a general idea of what **Team** X chooses to eat. It offers a handful of some of their favorite recipes from the not so healthy (but far from the worst) diet of Danny, to the fairly healthy eating habits of Inara, to the extreme, nutritional intake of Billy. Nutrition, like exercise, is a science. There are basic physiological rules that stay the same, regardless of diet. The foundation of proper nutrition never changes. It's the choices that form our habits – hence the outcome on our bodies and lives – that fluctuate.

The dilemma with food is that we need it to live, but our eating habits, or urges, are often the very things limiting our lives. Healthy eating habits don't just happen though. They are made by choice, again and again. To start, we recommend stocking your kitchen with things like apples, oranges, avocados, celery, raw nuts, etc. Then when you crave a snack you'll have better choices available. Just make them.

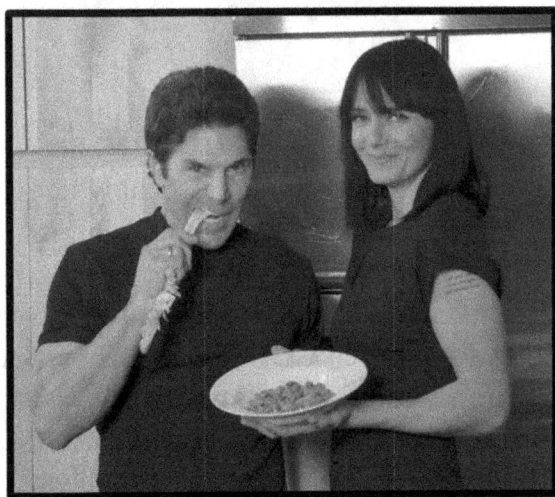

But unlike Billy, you may not crave celery like a rabid dog.

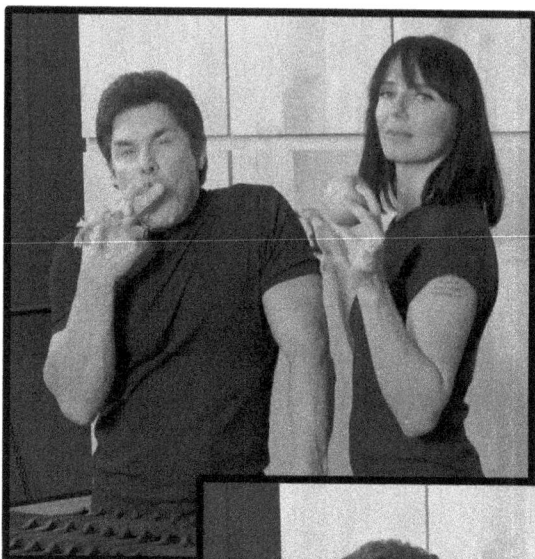

At least Billy's habits are good ones (albeit sometimes strangely expressed), while Inara chooses to be healthy <u>and</u> classy.

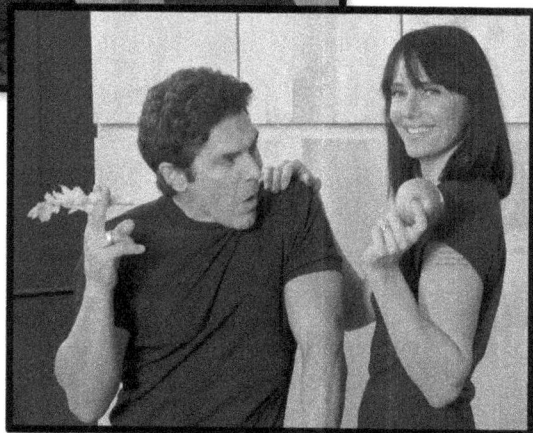

Know too, we are not saying you must give up things you love to eat. We are not saying you must eat like Billy or Inara (though probably not like Danny). Your eating habits are your choice. But if they aren't giving you a healthy, in-shape body, then maybe you should change them. It may not be easy to do, but it is that simple (see **GOOD CARBS vs BAD CARBS, Suggested Substitutions**, and **Recommended Vitamins and Supplements** at the end of this chapter for help in figuring it all out).

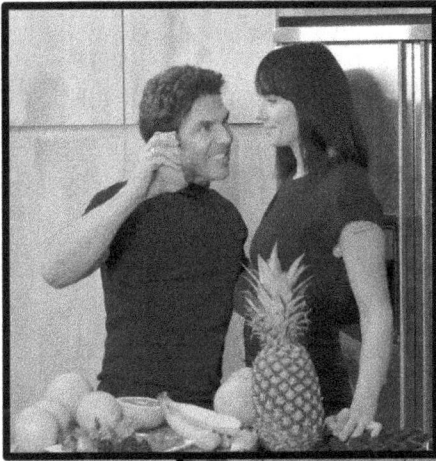

Though Billy is passionate about eating healthy, his methods of persuasion may be a bit forceful. Conversely, Inara chooses a more passive path of influence.

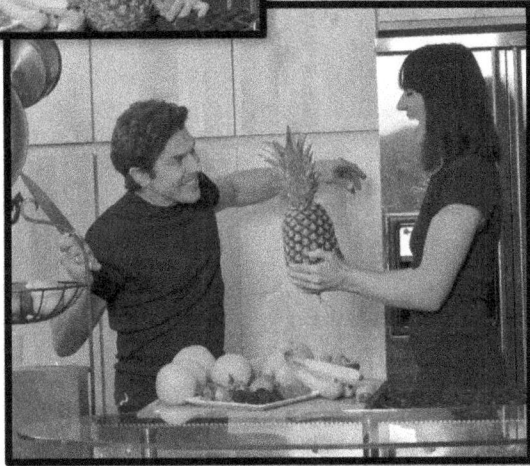

And certainly there are better and safer ways to slice a pineapple.

All this book can do is try to steer you to what we see as the right direction. Just please consider: if the main reason to eat is to live (and we submit it is), then you should eat accordingly.

The following recipes* offer a glimpse into some of the eating habits of **Team** X, with a few healthy (or at least healthier) crumbs to get you started.

*Don't be afraid to vary them to taste. **Team** X does.

— Billy's Diet —

There was a time when Billy ate candy bars and fries like everyone else. Additionally, let's just say he abused his body. Then, about thirty years ago, he morphed into being a "health nut" (or a "healthy nut"). The same addictive personality that placed him in harm's way early in his career, is the same fanatical force that drives him to what most people would consider, at present, a fairly-radical, mostly-raw diet. But it's hard to argue with the results.

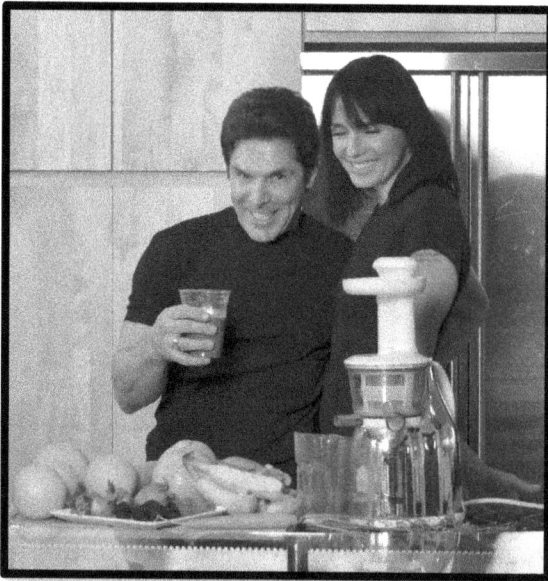

"I eat when I'm hungry, because that's the time to eat – when you're hungry, not because you smell or see food. Find your pleasure elsewhere. If it doesn't have value, don't eat it. Don't do it! We aren't dogs... usually... well sometimes." – Billy

Billy's Organic Protein Shake

2 scoops – SUNWARRIOR PROTEIN Warrior Blend
1 tbsp. – chia seeds*
1 tbsp. – coconut oil
5 drops (approx. or to taste) – vanilla Stevia
1 tsp. – cinnamon (Billy uses a lot more)
24 oz. – water or unsweetened almond milk (if ice
       is added, then add less liquid)

    Mix everything in a shaker and keep cold.
    Billy makes it daily in the morning, drinks half and
saves the rest for a snack later.

Optional additions:
    1 tsp. – Bentonite Clay**
    1 tsp. – powdered Ziolite***
    1 tbsp. – Vitamin C powder****

* provides 25-30 grams of protein
**absorbs toxins; flushes out kidneys and gall bladder
***eliminates heavy metals in the body
****antioxidant; promotes healthy skin, bones and
blood vessels

Billy's Organic Vegetable Juice

2-3 – large kale leaves
6 – celery stalks
1 – whole lemon (skin and all)
1 – whole apple (skin and all)
½ inch – ginger (or more)
1 – small cucumber (skin and all)
1 – small handful of parsley
1 – small handful of cilantro
1 – small handful of sprouts

Blend in juicer* and keep cold. Makes 16 to 24 oz. Billy tries to drink it daily.

* Low RPM juicers leave more fiber in the juice, which helps regulate the fructose level. They yield a better tasting juice that lasts longer. Plus they're quieter.

Billy's Misc. Organic Drinks*

16 oz. – ice-cold water
1 – whole squeezed lemon

Optional additions:
    1 packet – Stevia
    raw apple-cider vinegar
    1 tsp. – quality powdered ginger

*substitute for **Billy's Organic Protein Shake** or **Billy's Organic Vegetable Juice**

Billy's Fast, Organic Guacamole*

1 – avocado
1 – handful of cherry tomatoes
garlic powder (to taste)
1 tbsp. – lemon or lime juice
cayenne pepper (to taste)
cumin (to taste)
1/8 cup – cilantro (finely chopped)

Mash the avocado with a fork. Cut the tomatoes in half and mix into the avocado along with the garlic powder, lemon/lime juice, cayenne pepper, cumin and cilantro.
Best eaten fresh.

Optional addition:
¼ cup – onion (finely chopped; Billy doesn't use)

*an excellent spread (see **Billy's Organic Wrap**)

Billy's Organic Broccolini

½ lb. (approx. 12 stalks) – broccolini
6 cloves – minced garlic
1/8 cup – olive oil
¼ cup – water
¼ cup – fresh basil (chopped)
¼ bunch – fresh cilantro (chopped)
cayenne powder (to taste)
sea salt (optional; to taste)

Optional addition:
    organic, raw sauerkraut (to taste)

Cut broccolini into bitesize pieces (including stalk).

In large skillet, heat olive oil and minced garlic for 2 minutes on low. Add broccolini and water. Cover and simmer for an additional 1 minute. Add sea salt and warmed sauerkraut if desired.

Billy likes it hot or cold (but then Billy also runs hot or cold).

Billy's Organic Vegetable Medley

4 bunches – broccolini
1 lb. – Italian tomatoes (canned or fresh*)
½ tube – organic Trader Joe's tomato paste
6 cloves – garlic** (minced)
¼ cup – fresh parsley** (finely chopped)
¼ cup – fresh cilantro** (finely chopped)
cumin (to taste; Billy uses a lot)
¼ cup – water
olive oil

Optional additions:
   3-4 – fresh jalapeño peppers (sliced)
   ¼ cup – onions (finely chopped; Billy doesn't use)

If using jalapeños, cut off top, remove seeds and slice into strips. Sautee covered, in a large, frying pan (add onions if desired) with a small amount of olive oil. Remove from pan.

Add garlic and broccolini to pan. Pour in water, with enough olive oil to cover. Sautee covered until fork tender and water has been absorbed. Mix in tomatoes and tomato paste (and jalapeños and onions). Simmer covered for about 3 minutes.

Stir in parsley and cilantro. Sprinkle with cumin.

* if using fresh tomatoes, steam first, then peel
**Trader Joes has pre-packed garlic, onions and many frozen herbs that are great when in a hurry.

<u>Billy's Organic Wrap</u>

4 tbsp. – **Billy's Fast, Organic Guacamole**
1 large leaf – collard greens*
3-4 stalks – broccolini
2 tbsp. – raw hummus w/cayenne pepper**
2 tbsp. – fresh parsley (finely chopped)
2 tbsp. – fresh cilantro (finely chopped)

    Spread **Billy's Fast, Organic Guacamole** on a raw collard greens leaf. Spread with hummus. Then add a layer of cooked broccolini***. Season with parsley and cilantro. Roll the leaf and eat fresh.
    You may want more than one.

Optional additions****:
    Billy's Organic Vegetable Medley
    red bell pepper (chopped or sliced)

*Billy sometimes substitutes with a brown rice tortilla, though it's not as healthy. It depends on how lazy he's feeling or if he feels he needs some quick carbs.
**available at health food stores
***see recipe for **Billy's Organic Broccolini**
****for those eating meat or seafood you could add chicken breast, lean beef, pork loin, shrimp, etc.; Billy rarely, if ever, eats meat or seafood.

Billy's Comfort Foods and Snacks:
Billy's Organic Protein Shake
Billy's Organic Broccolini (hot or cold)
Cashews and Brazil nuts
1 spoonful (or 2) – organic cashew/almond butter
Smashed raspberries and cashew/almond butter
Sweet potato with cinnamon (maybe coconut oil)
Avocados
Cinnamon (on just about everything sweet)
Hummus (on just about everything else)

Billy Never Eats or Drinks:
bread; pastry; pasta; white rice; white potatoes
sugar; bananas (that could change); alcohol

Billy's Vitamins and Supplements (partial list)
Omega 3 fish oil
K2
D3
Zinc
Magnesium

Billy's uses food as his basic platform of vitamins and minerals, which changes constantly, depending on what he feels he needs at the moment.

"Only crazy people do the stuff I do. I get my kicks on raspberries sprinkled with cinnamon. Plus it cleanses. It's an ongoing process. The point is, you can't beat nature." – Billy

— Inara's Diet —

Inara's diet would probably be considered by most to be a healthy alternative without being drastic. That's not saying it's better, just that it might be an easier one to follow and swallow.

Inara eats few carbs, but does indulge in things like brown rice pasta and brown rice tortillas. She often enjoys a steak with broccoli or string beans (with a tiny touch of butter) and a sweet potato (plain, no butter). Other than that her choices are fairly simple.

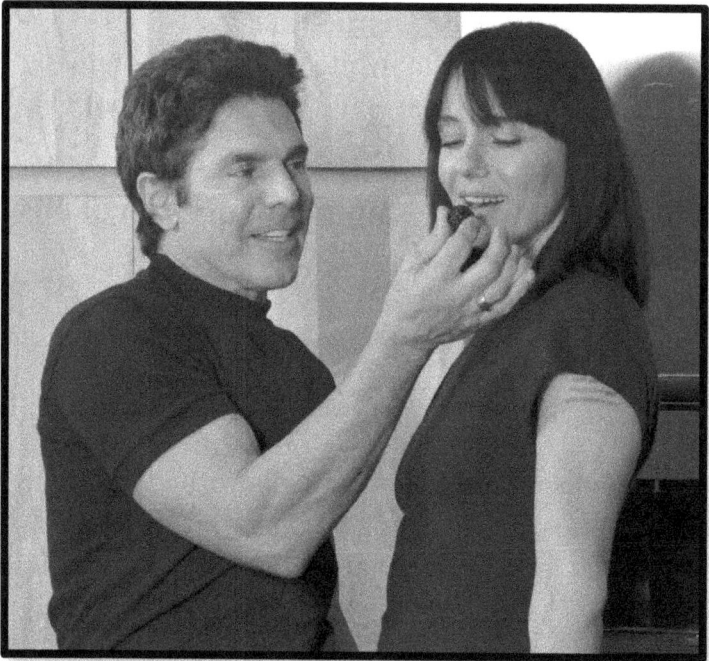

"Billy isn't above force-feeding anything from food to philosophy, but I'm not above biting." – Inara

Inara's Organic Breakfast Smoothie

2 large leaves – kale
1 scoop – vanilla protein powder
1 cup – water
1 cup – ice
1 tbsp. – almond butter
1 – peeled banana

Blend kale, protein powder, water, banana and almond butter first. Then add ice and blend until fairly smooth. That's it.

Best to drink it right away. Makes about 16 ounces.

Inara's Organic Energy Juice

1 – small beet
2 – small cucumbers
1 – large red apple
5 – carrots
½ inch – ginger
1 tbsp. – lemon juice

Using a juicer, combine the beet, cucumbers, apple, carrots and ginger.

Mix lemon juice into the blend with a spoon.

Drink right away or chill for later. Makes about 12-16 ounces.

<u>Inara's Organic Banana Wrap</u>

1 – extra-large flour tortilla
1 – banana
almond butter

Heat tortilla in a dry pan until slightly browned. Remove from pan and spread with desired amount of almond butter. Place the banana on the tortilla and roll.

Best eaten warm, although Inara also likes it cold.

<u>Inara's Organic Egg Fold</u>

1 – extra-large flour tortilla
2 – eggs
2 strips – uncured bacon

Cook the bacon to desired crispiness and use the bacon grease* to fry (or scramble) the eggs.

Before the eggs are finished, heat the tortilla in a dry pan until slightly browned. Lay the heated tortilla on a plate and place the cooked egg and bacon on one half. Season to taste (Inara adds a splash of Cholula hot sauce) and fold in half while the tortilla is still pliable.

*if bacon or bacon grease isn't used, substitute with a small amount of olive oil.

Inara's Beef Casserole

1 lb. – ground beef and pork mix
1 lb. – brown rice pasta
1 cup – chopped onion
a pinch of ground sea salt
2 tbsp. – chili powder*
1 tbsp. – cumin*
1-2 cups – spaghetti sauce**

Boil pasta to desired consistency.

While pasta is cooking, splash onion with some olive oil and cook on a pan until starts to get clear. Remove onions, and brown meat until thoroughly cooked. Drain excess grease and add onions and rest of ingredients, including cooked and drained pasta. Cover and simmer for ten minutes.

Add extra seasonings to taste and extra sauce if needed (Inara uses very little sauce).

*Inara often uses Russian spices instead and/or in addition (all names written in Russian, so good luck).
**Inara uses any Classico sauce that has no added sugar.

Inara's Comfort Foods and Snacks:
Too much coffee (with half 'n' half ; no sweetener)
An occasional glass of wine
Trader Joe's trail mix (nuts, cranberries & seeds)
Dill pickles
A slice of pie on Thanksgiving and Christmas
½ of a Napoleon on a few birthdays
Occasionally, Trader Joes dark chocolate
Sometimes, Think or Atkins bars for a boost
Is known to snack on Ikea's sugarless cookies

Inara Never (almost never) Eats or Drinks:
bread; pastry; white potatoes; sugary things; carbonated beverages

Inara's Vitamins and Supplements:
Omega 3
Multi-vitamins (though Billy recommends not to)
Vitamin C

– Danny's Diet –

Danny is an observer of healthy eating, which means he has no problem watching others do it. He does try to eat better than he used to, but as said earlier, his diet may not be one to be followed. We suggest you gauge your diet against his to see how you either might improve or are already doing better.

Danny doesn't eat meat but isn't a strict Vegetarian because he still eats seafood. Some of his favorite meals used to be meatloaf with mashed potatoes and gravy, pork loin and potato stew, veal scaloppini, lasagna – all staples of his mother's cooking growing up (along with every pie, cake, cookie and bread under the sun). Now he enjoys shrimp, salmon, eggplant parmesan, guacamole, tomatoes, white and sweet potatoes, broccoli, green beans, corn and various other cooked vegetables all with too much butter, a lot of pepper, but no salt.

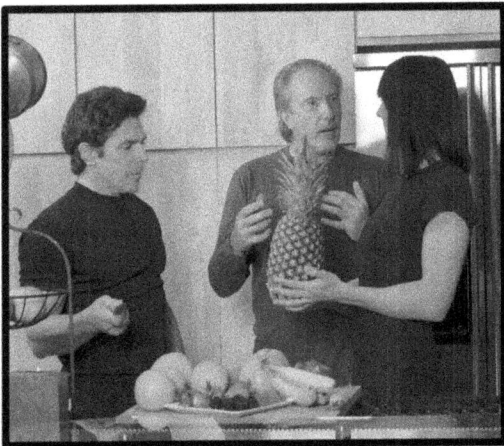

With a knife in hand, Billy isn't sure whether he should cut the pineapple or Danny, for some of his questionable food choices.

Danny's Organic Smoothie*

½ cup – raw almonds (2 – Trader Joe's handful-bags)
1 ½ cups – unsweetened coconut milk
1 tbsp. – raw, unsweetened almond butter
1 tbsp. – cocoa powder
1 cup – ice (the more ice, the thicker the smoothie)
1 (or 2) – pitted dates

   Pour almond milk into blender. Add almonds, cocoa powder, dates and blend. Add almond butter and blend again. Add ice and blend until desired smoothness. Makes about 16 ounces.

*amounts are approximate; vary to taste.

Danny's Organic Energy Drink

1 – grapefruit (peeled and sectioned)
1 – orange (peeled and sectioned)
2 – green apples
1 – slice of pineapple (approx. ½ cup)
1 – small cucumber
1 – long carrot
1 inch – ginger (or more; Danny likes the kick)

   Juice the grapefruit, orange, apples, pineapple, cucumber, carrot and ginger. Strain off the foam.
   Drink right away or chill for later (about 16 oz).

Danny's Favorite Vegetable Chili

¾ cup – olive oil

2 – medium-size zucchinis (cut into ½ in. cubes)

2 – medium-size yellow onions (cut into ½ in. cubes)

4 cloves – garlic (finely chopped)

2 – large, red bell peppers (diced into ¼ in pieces)

1 can (35 oz.) – Italian plum tomatoes (<u>undrained</u>)

1 ½ lb. – fresh plum tomatoes (cut into 1 in. cubes)

2 tbsp. – chili powder

1 tbsp. – ground cumin

1 tbsp. – dried basil

1 tbsp. – dried oregano

½ cup – fresh Italian parsley (chopped)

½ cup – fresh dill (chopped)

2 tbsp. – freshly ground black pepper

1 tsp. – salt (optional; Danny doesn't add it)

1 tsp. – fennel seeds

2 tbsp. – tamed jalapeño peppers (chopped)

1 cup – canned black beans (drained)

1 cup – canned garbanzo beans/chick-peas (drained)

Sauté zucchini in ½ cup olive oil, under medium heat until tender. Transfer zucchini from oil to a large pot. Add remaining oil and sauté onions, red pepper, and garlic (low heat) until tender. Add to pot with oil.

Add canned and fresh tomatoes, oregano, parsley, cumin, chili powder, fennel, basil, pepper, and salt. Simmer for 30 minutes. Stir in black beans, garbanzo beans, dill and lemon juice. Cook for 15 minutes more.

Add favorite hot sauce to taste (Danny adds tons).

<u>Danny's Comfort Foods and Snacks</u>:
> pizza (with red/green peppers and extra cheese)
> Popeye's popcorn shrimp
> fried zucchini
> french fries
> potato chips
> chips and salsa
> all kinds of nuts
> occasional sweets
> occasional can of Fresca
> way too much cheese
> too much butter
> popcorn (at the movies)

<u>Danny Never Eats or Drinks</u>:
> meat; added salt (except on French fries); alcohol;
> coffee; any liquid with caffeine (except an
> occasional hot chocolate, a rare tea or
> an extremely rare soda)

<u>Danny's Vitamins and Supplements</u>:
> Do nuts count? (*"Actually, they do."* – Billy)

* * * * * * * * *

GOOD CARBS vs BAD CARBS

There are three types of carbohydrates: sugars, starches and fiber. They all have different functions, but exactly how they affect our health is a matter of much discussion and varying opinions. Our simple version is: natural sugar is good, while processed sugar is bad; food containing whole grains is good and food containing refined grains is bad. But to really understand their place in a healthy diet we strongly suggest you research the matter on your own. It all has to do with blood sugar, it's absorption into the body and all sorts of processes that are truly too involved for this book. We'll give you the basics only. And while opinions vary as to whether you should count carbs or calories, our thought is, if you stick to good carbs and avoid the bad, your waistline especially will thank you.

So, to begin with, when sugar enters the body it is turned into glucose. Our bodies then produce insulin to manage the distribution of the glucose – not too much or too little. That's why the right amount of good carbs is important. The major difference between good carbs and bad carbs is that good carbs, also known as slow carbs, usually don't result in a rapid rise in blood sugar (the glucose) followed by a fast drop in energy; energy that we need for things like exercising. Glucose is also needed for muscle and tissue repair. Bad carbs, on the other hand, or fast carbs, are prone to spiking our blood sugar causing insulin to increase as it tries to manage the glucose.

Sometimes we may find that we need a rush when our energy is low, which is why when we eat a candy bar, it's like an instant shot of glucose and our insulin reacts accordingly. We aren't telling you to do that, just what happens when you do. However, an apple will generally give you the same results and should keep your insulin levels more in check.

Insulin is a hormone created in the pancreas that when released, signals muscle, fat, and liver cells in the body to absorb glucose (the ingested sugar) from the bloodstream to be used for energy. And when the body has more glucose than it needs insulin stores it in the liver to be used later. It also tells the liver when to release glucose. Good carbs enable insulin to do its job, while bad carbs inhibit its proper function by overloading the amount of glucose in the body.

So, again, the simple version of choosing the right carbs is: choose carbs that are high in fiber, contain whole grains and are not too high in starch. And stick to the natural sugar found in fruit, vegetables and yes, dairy. Fruits and vegetables do contain fast carbs, however their fiber content is also high, making absorption into the body more like slow carbs.

The main problems with carbs are the starches and sugars they contain. So, a good rule of thumb is, *choose sugar that comes from natural sources and choose starches that contain whole grains without a high starch content.* Just remember this is only the simple version, with a breakdown as follows:

SUGARS

The two main types of sugar are:

<u>Natural sugars</u> – fruits, vegetables and dairy.

Natural sugars are exactly what they sound like – natural. They are found in fruits and vegetables (fructose) and milk and other dairy products (lactose).

<u>Processed sugars</u> – added to foods like canned fruit, breakfast cereals, etc., with names such as table sugar, brown sugar, powdered sugar, molasses and others.

Processed sugars are found in just about everything manufactured, because it tastes good and makes us want more, healthiness withstanding.

As we mentioned earlier, regardless of the type of sugar, when it's ingested, it's turned into glucose to be absorbed into the blood. Processed sugars are absorbed quickly and cause spikes in our blood sugar levels resulting in a high insulin release. Put simply, that screws up our whole system, hence the unnatural highs and lows they produce.

The natural sugars in fruit and vegetables – while sweeter than processed sugars and almost as detrimental in large quantities – have the advantage of the fiber they contain, in edible skin and seeds; the same fiber that has been removed from the fructose in processed fruit juices and dried fruit. Fiber slows the absorption of glucose, which keeps our insulin at a more normal level.

Lactose on the other hand is broken down in the intestines. But for those who are intolerant, it unfortunately sits in the stomach causing gas, bloating, cramps and diarrhea. If you find that to be your problem, you can try lactose-free dairy or just don't consume dairy at all*. And the jury is still out on whether reduced fat is healthier than whole milk. Again, your own research may be required.

*Just so you know, Billy eats no dairy at all, Inara uses half & half, no milk and rarely butter and Danny hardly ever drinks milk but eats a lot of other dairy, especially cheese. You decide what's best. However, we suggest you lean toward following Billy or Inara.

STARCHES

Starch provides three absorbable forms of sugar – glucose, fructose and galactose – that are derived from plant matter.

Vegetables and dried beans that are high in starch include: peas, corn, lima beans, white potatoes, lentils, pinto beans, kidney beans, black-eyed peas and more.

Grains high in starch include: oats, barley and rice. Grains, however, are made up of three parts: bran (fiber, B vitamins and minerals); germ (loaded with nutrients, essential fatty acids and E vitamins); and endosperm (pure starch). So, when eating grains, stick with whole grain foods that contain all three parts. Refined grain foods only contain endosperm.

FIBER

Fiber is found in plant foods such as fruits, vegetables, whole grains, nuts and legumes. It is the indigestible part of the plant which means most of it passes through your digestive system and takes things with it, which is a good thing. Additionally, high fiber diets are thought to reduce cholesterol levels. But it's hard to get enough fiber, so as long as it's in the good carb category, eat all you can.

Some good sources of fiber include:

1) Beans (especially black beans, kidney beans, pinto beans, garbanzo beans and lentils) and legumes (members of the pea family)

2) Vegetables and Fruit (especially those with edible skin and edible seeds)

3) Whole grain foods (some pasta, some cereals, some breads – though Billy never eats them).

4) Nuts (almonds, peanuts and walnuts – but stick with unsalted or at least with sea salt and preferably raw).

* * * * * * * * * * *

In summary, stay away from refined grains (generally the whiter the grain, the lower the fiber) and do your best to totally remove processed sugars from your diet.

To give you an idea of what's best, following is an abbreviated list of good carbs and bad carbs, divided into food groups, to help you make a better choice.

<u>Good Carbs</u>	<u>Bad Carbs</u>
most all vegetables	potatoes (and other white vegetables)
fresh fruit	bananas, pineapples and grapes (though not actually bad, they are all high in fructose
whole grains	anything white or made with refined grains
most all nuts and seeds especially raw and unsalted almonds, peanuts, brazil nuts, cashews), soy beans and beans/pea family (eat in moderation)	nuts with coatings and corn nuts; <u>sweetened</u> peanut butter, cashew butter or almond butter
some dairy* (whole milk, cream, cheese, sour cream, butter	ice cream, sweetened yogurt, reduced fat milk or skim milk
whole grain crackers, pickles, olives	potato chips, pretzels, corn chips, popcorn, candy, cookies, rice cakes, granola bars, crackers

*just don't overdo it

* * * * * * * * *

Suggested Substitutions:

Sodas.................seltzer water; plain water or
                     water with added lemon juice
                     or Sweet Leaf brand flavorings
Bread.................brown rice tortillas
Milk....................almond milk or rice milk
Sugar.................Stevia brand sweetener
Salt..................... raw Himalayan sea salt or
                     imitation salt (if you must have it)
Butter................olive oil (cooking); coconut oil
                     (cooking or as a spread)
Salad dressing....Tomato (marinara) sauce or
                     hummus

Recommended Vitamins* and Supplements:

Again, the best source of vitamins and minerals is
from the original source: food. But until you get that
figured out (it's an ongoing process that even Billy
keeps changing) the following is a good start.

Omega 3
K2
D3
B complex (maybe; especially if Vegetarian/Vegan)
Zinc
Selenium
Magnesium

*Multi-vitamins are not needed with the right food

> *"When something is important enough, you do it even if the odds are not in your favor."*
> – Elon Musk

9   MORE ABOUT *Team* X

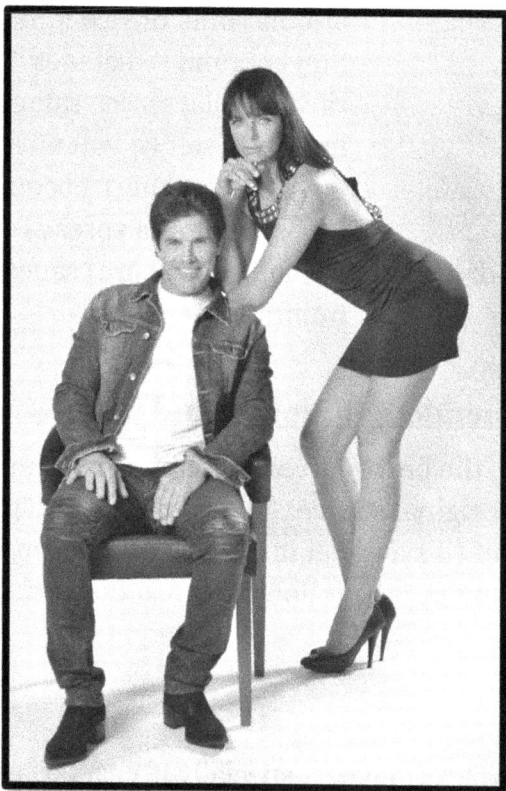

    Team X isn't perfect. They're always trying to be better, though fighting beliefs about age isn't easy. But Billy is a fitness fanatic and Inara is driven to excel (even Danny is mindful), and the following life choices are how they got to where they are in this book.

294

BILLY NUZZO

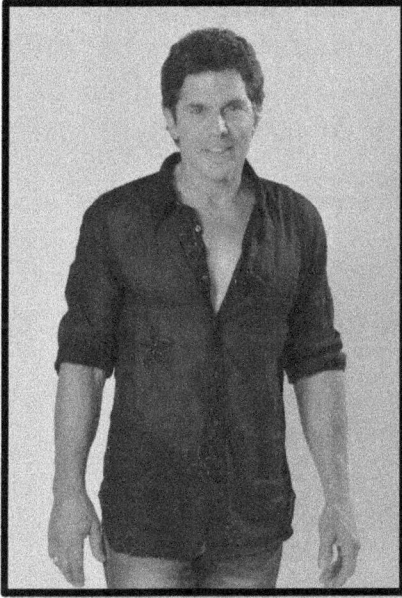

Billy is a lifetime Fitness Guru, a Nutrition Expert, a career Craft Service Chef to the stars, an accomplished guitar player and most importantly, a Single Dad (with a little one). Growing up in New Haven, Connecticut, Billy comes from a long line of restaurateurs and dubious "tough guys". Billy's culinary talents have satisfied palates, the likes of Sean Connery, Ted Danson, Jerry Seinfeld, Chris Rock, William Shatner, Julia Louis Dryfuss and Will Ferrell among many others on such productions as Seinfeld, All in the Family, Star Trek, Becker, Dr. Phil, American Pie, Entertainment Tonight and a whole lot more. He's known on set, not just for his cooking, but for his more-than-outspoken personality, offering solicited and unsolicited advice on everything from the right way to exercise, to healthy eating, to proper parenting, to "what's wrong with you people?" and how to fix it. So, at 69, he knows what he's talking about, but to benefit you have to listen.

Billy works out for 30-45 minutes every day, primarily at home, for the purpose of muscle maintenance. He's a big fan of the chin-up bar, push-ups and the stairs. He also bike rides about three times a week for round trips of usually forty-five miles or more.

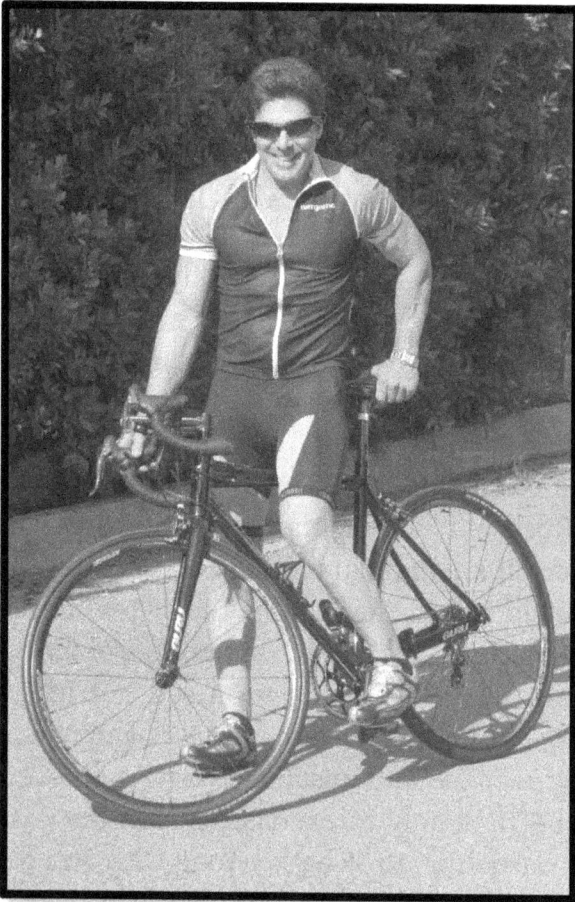

"There's nothing like seeing a mountain ahead of you and knowing, 'I can do that.' It's amazing." - Billy

Resume

Billy's Formal Education:

The Emilio Borelli Acting Studio
(Cold Reading Acting)

Dr. Jane Major
("Breakthrough Parenting")

Sous Chef
(apprenticed for Hollywood Chef, Adel Chagar)

Karen Voight Studio
(The Art of Teaching Fitness)

ISSA Sports Institute –
Certified Personal Trainer
(Sports Injury Prevention, Sports Nutrition
and CPR-AED)

UCLA
Quinnipiac University
University of New Haven

Billy's Informal Education:

Dad's backhand
Working at the family restaurant
"Uncle" Dickies Cadillac Lessons
A.A.
Lead Guitarist (my rock 'n' roll days): "Bad Nuzzo"
Getting married/divorced
Becoming a SINGLE DAD (with a little one)

Billy's Accomplishments/Awards:

Special Judge – "Guess Who's Ass" segment:
"The Donny and Marie Show"

Personal Information

Billy's Diet (BASICALLY RAW)*:
> Breakfast – Billy's choices are usually:
>> **Billy's Organic Protein Shake**;
>> **Billy's Organic Vegetable Juice**;
>>> & some very unpleasant tasting things
> Lunch – at no set time, an avocado salad or a raw
>> hummus platter or more protein drink
> Dinner – Billy eats the same things over and over
> Snacks – not big on snacks
> Drinks – water or raw beverages
> Vitamins – too numerous to list
> Guilty Pleasures – his food is too boring for guilt

* see **THINGS WE EAT** – **Billy's Diet** for examples

Billy's Favorite Exercises:
> Billy "enjoys" climbing stairs and leg lifts on the chin-up bar, but he actually enjoys bike riding.

Billy's Basic Philosophy:
> *"The trap is thinking you have all the time in the world to start exercising. You don't. The goal is to be able to look in the mirror and say, "I'd f#@$ me".*

Billy's Contact Info:
> billynuzzopresents.com
> nuzzo.billy@gmail.com

INARA LOPETAITE

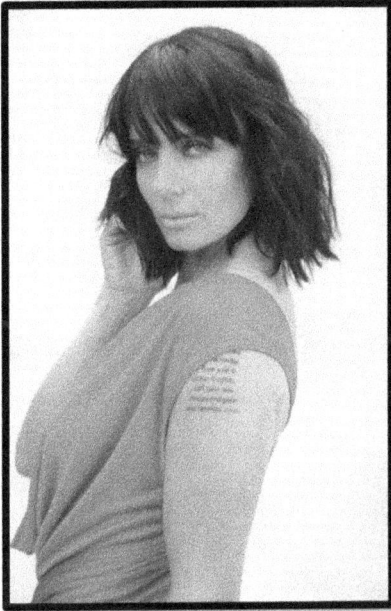

Inara is a former runway/print Model, a Beauty Competition Winner and a published Author (of original poems), from Panevezys, Lithuania. Having spent her first 30 years in Eastern Europe (14 of those in the Soviet Union), Inara knows what it means to never give up. Now, as a Hollywood Make-Up Artist for fashion and beauty, a licensed Esthetician for celebrity clients (since 2017) and a 43-year-old mother of teenage twins, she also knows the importance of effort and persistence in achieving your career goals.

After spending her early years before a camera, she is presently enjoying being behind the scenes as well. Although, at the click of a shutter, she's ready to step back into a Model's high heels or simply strike a pose.

Inara was always conscious of keeping fit during her Pageant days (most recently as Mrs. Lithuania in the 2011 Mrs. World Competition), but it wasn't until 2013 that she started to seriously train.

Inara tries to work out for roughly one hour, three to five days a week. For her, the gym is a refuge from her busy schedule at home and with clients.

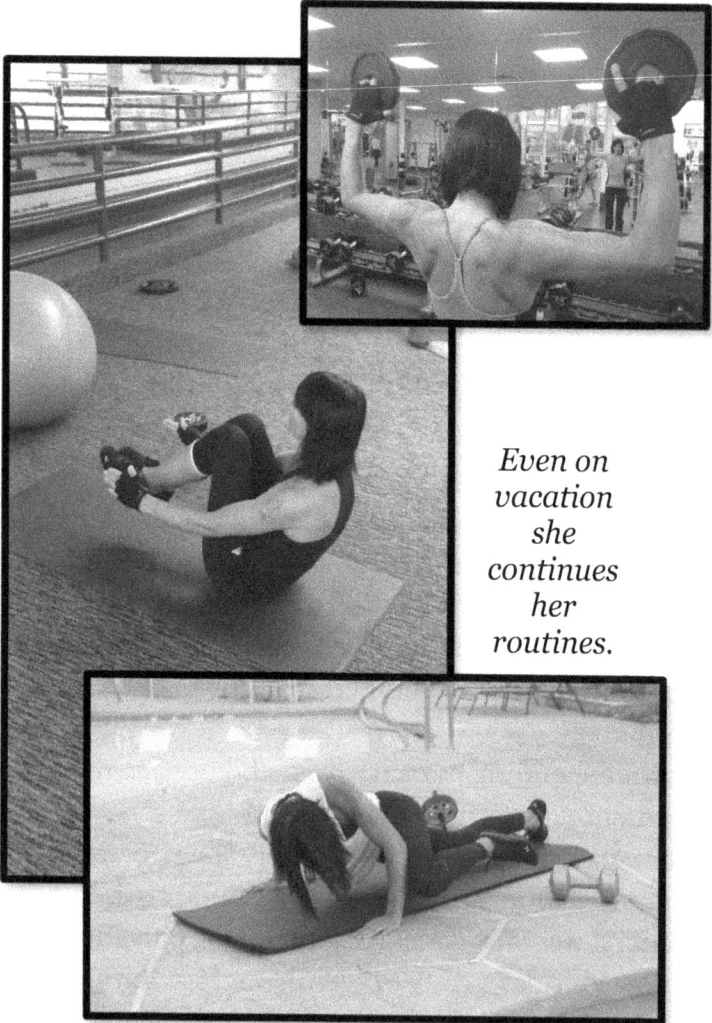

Even on vacation she continues her routines.

"I'm invigorated when I work out. It makes me feel bright." – Inara

Resume

Inara's Formal Education:
Yakov Gershkovich Aesthetics School, Int'l.
(face sculpting and lifting techniques)
LA Trade Technical College, Los Angeles, CA
(licensed Esthetician)
Studio Make-Up Academy, Hollywood, CA
(Beauty and SFX)
Cambridge Institute, Copenhagen, Denmark
(English)
Niels Brock University, Copenhagen, Denmark
(International Business)
Andrisiuno Bus. School, Panevezys, Lithuania
(Business)

Inara's Informal Education:
Modeling for print and runway
Working as a Freelance Make-Up Artist
Training at the gym
Self-taught Oil Painter
Mother of twins

Inara's Accomplishments/Awards:
L'Oréal contract at age 14
Published Author: *"Love Has No Price"*
("Most Beautiful Book" – 2008; in Lithuania)
Miss Resort 1996 (3rd Place and Miss Photogenic)
Miss Resort 1997 (3rd Place and People's Choice)
Miss Region 1997 (1st Place)
Mrs. US Globe 2010 (3rd Place)

Personal Information

Inara's Diet (BASICALLY HEALTHY/LOW CARB):

Breakfast – Oatmeal with fruit or 2 eggs or
a protein drink

Lunch – usually a fruit and vegetable drink/
smoothie or a salad

Dinner – generally lean meat, chicken or fish,
brown rice (or brown rice pasta),
black beans and vegetables

Snacks – a spoonful of organic almond butter,
raw nuts, apples or bananas

Drinks – water, protein drinks and raw drinks

Guilty Pleasures – a rare Margarita; occasional
wine or Fresca; some sugar-free
chocolate; some pie (birthdays,
Thanksgiving and Christmas)

Inara's Favorite Exercises:
Squats, lunges and whole body routines

Inara's Basic Philosophy:
"In a few words it's, 'Daryti tai kas jums atrodo taisingai.' Translated to English it means, 'Follow your own truth'. I wear it on my arm... literally."

Inara's Contact Info:
inara.lopetaite@yahoo.com

DANIEL AKIN

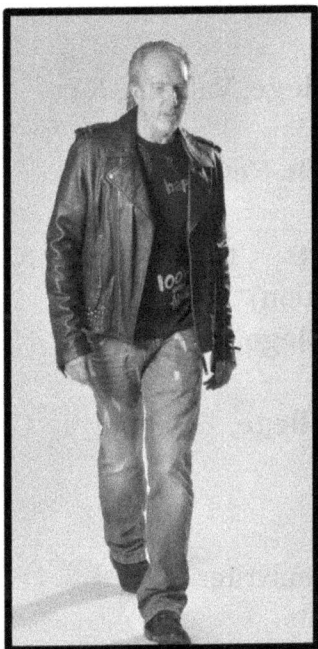

Danny is a Screenwriter from Back-East (New York). He is more of a fitness enthusiast than an expert. However, he is an avid "Conceptualizer" and was compelled – by the results of Billy and Inara's workout ethics – to capture what they do in written and visual form. He figured that others could benefit from their motivation and guidance. So, he hefted a pen and along with Billy and Inara created, The Zero-Minute Workout.

When he's not writing, Danny is usually busy "researching" (all tax deductible) or doing something he doesn't want to do. That said, he has also been a Production Assistant, an Assistant Camera Operator, a Production Manager, an Editor, a Director/Producer (black comedy videos starring, Billy; and more) and even a Studio Driver. And he's fairly handy with hand tools, which were only needed for this project once.

While Billy and Inara are the true backbone of **Team** X, Danny's role is more like that of its middle finger... along with its index finger and thumb. And as a Writer, he is only as good as the material that first inspired him: Billy Nuzzo and Inara Lopetaite.

Resume

<u>Danny's Formal Education</u>:

Westchester Comm. College, Valhalla, NY
(Advertising)

School of Social Research, New York, NY
(Screenwriting)

School of Visual Arts, New York, NY
(Film and Video Production)

Jamestown Comm. College, Jamestown, NY
(Video Production)

Connecticut State College, Danbury, CT
(Secondary Education)

<u>Danny's Informal Education</u>:

Working as a Freelance Screenwriter
Reading and fixing bad scripts
Copying my Father's life ethics
Forming Andyland Concepts, Inc.
Moving out to California with my best friend

<u>Danny's Accomplishments/Awards</u>:

Produced/Directed – *Single Dad (with a little one)*
                                         starring Billy Nuzzo
Created/retailed for Andyland Concepts, Inc. –
    Portable Properties: *"Affordable Real Estate"*
                                    Genuine Land (in a box);
    Land-by-the-Inch;
    and *Dirt Cheap Land*
Certified – "Master Monster Maker" (at age 10)

Personal Information

Danny's Diet* (PESCETARIAN):
  Breakfast – Oatmeal with fruit or 3 eggs or
                    sometimes an almond smoothie
  Lunch – at best, an almond smoothie; otherwise
                    probably something he shouldn't eat
  Dinner – seafood; fried zucchini; potato and eggs;
                    corn; cheese; crackers; occasional pasta
  Snacks – Atkin's coconut bars, various fruit or
                    Spanish peanuts
  Drinks – generally water; sometimes Fresca
  Vitamins – not enough, which means none
  Guilty Pleasures – French fries; pizza; Mexican
                    food; numerous bad things

Danny's Favorite Exercises:
  Racquetball (but not good); swimming; hiking

Danny's Basic Philosophy:
  Row, row, row your boat, gently down the stream.
  Merrily, merrily, merrily, merrily...
  Life is but a dream.

Danny's Contact Info:
  TheScriptDoc.com
  twitter.com/TheScriptDoc
  danakin@sbcglobal.net

*Pescetarian aside, Danny's diet isn't recommended.

                    * * * * * * * * *

If you take nothing else away from this book, always be thinking, "What exercise can I do right now? How can I turn what I'm doing, this very moment, into an Xer-task?" That's the whole idea.

Thanks for reading. And remember, the rest of your life starts this instant. Use your minutes wisely.

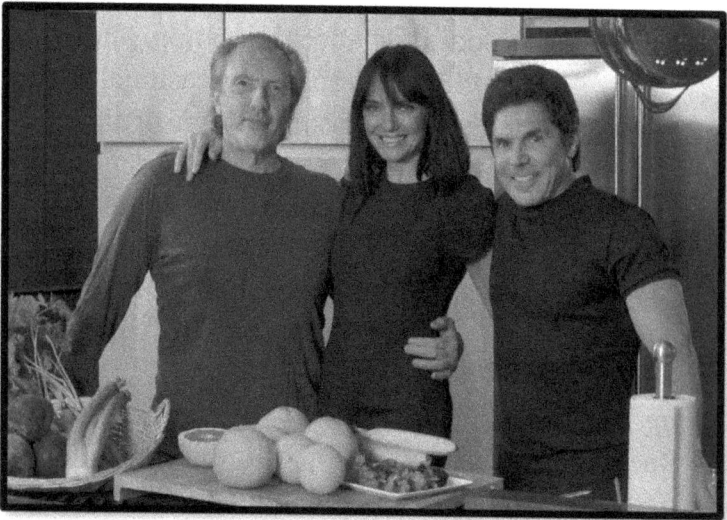

Sincerely,

Team X

Billy Nuzzo and Inara Lopetaite

(with Daniel Akin)

> *"It does not matter how slowly you go so long as you do not stop."* – Confucius

AFTERWORD

We started this project in June of 2014. At that time, Billy was still 65, Inara had just turned 39 and Danny was almost 62. As of this writing in June of 2018, Billy is 69, Inara is 43 and Danny is turning 66. All of the pictures in this book were taken in 2014 except those specifically noted as taken in 2017. We dare say you probably wouldn't have noticed the difference unless we told you (except maybe a little gray on Danny). Things were never meant to take this long, but they did. We never gave up on finishing this work, though there were certainly many times when that's what we wanted to do.

We offer these pages to you as a testament of perseverance and the sincere belief that you, too, can reach your individual fitness destinations. The thing is, life doesn't stop and wait for you to catch up. It keeps going. So, take charge and the circumstances, the condition and the quality of your being will follow.

Team X is more than just a name. An **X er-task** is more than a clever combination of words. And The Zero-Minute Workout is more than a unique idea. It's a way of life that's achievable by anyone who takes the time (the time you already have) to live it. You *can* succeed! Start today! Don't give up! Never stop! And be well. Always.   307

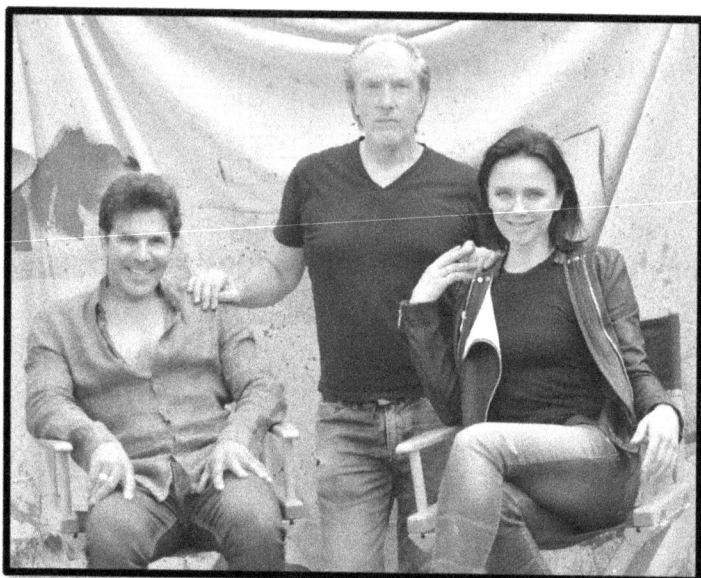

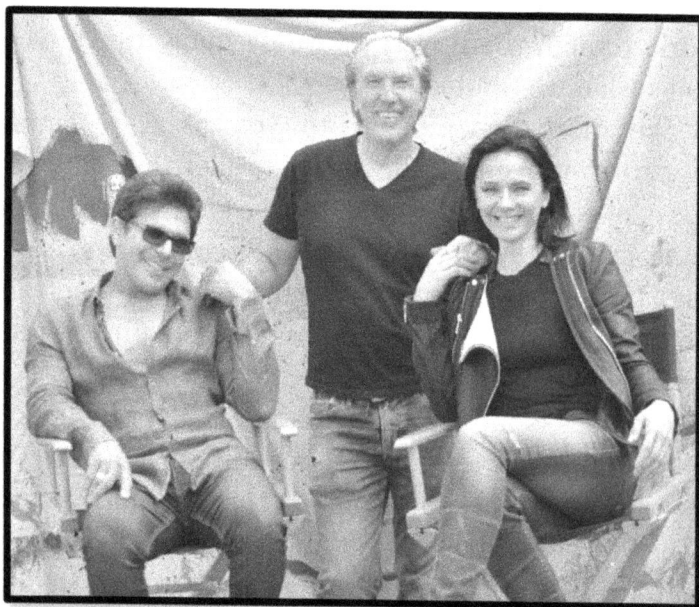

Pictures taken 2017

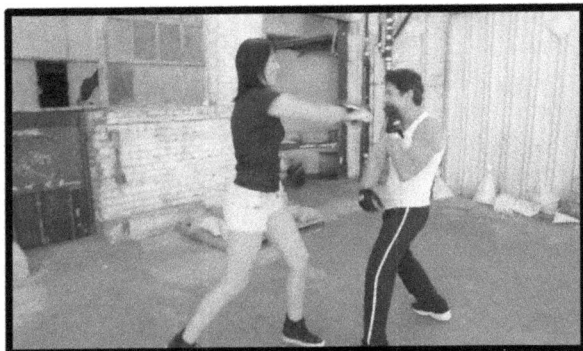

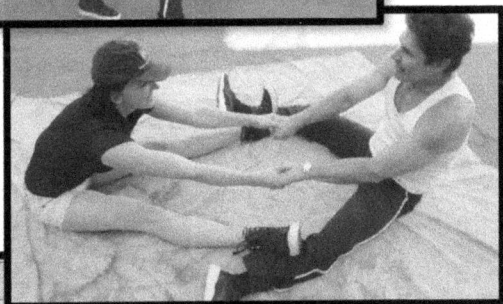

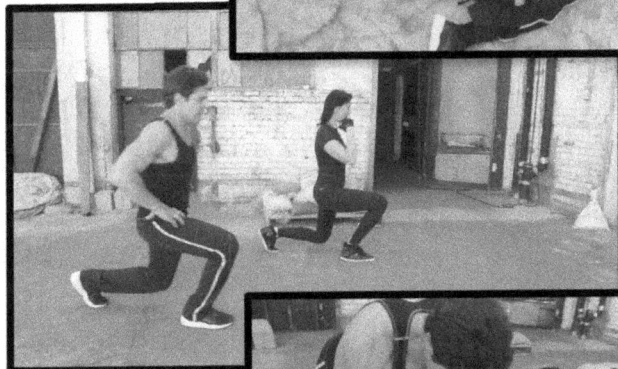

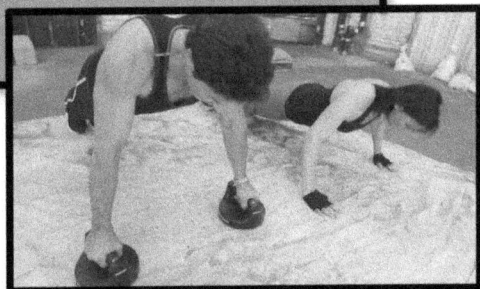

Pictures taken 2017 from promo videos
by Miguel Blake & Greta Tuckute